FROM
THIS DAY
FORWARD

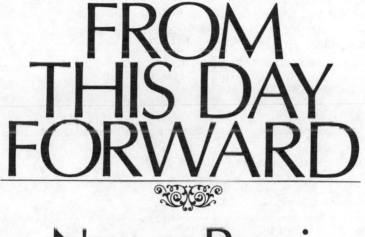

FROM
THIS DAY
FORWARD

Nancy Rossi

Times
BOOKS

In order to protect the privacy of certain individuals involved in this story, some names have been changed.

The quotations on pages 210 and 267 are from *The Complete Poems of Emily Dickinson*, edited by Thomas H. Johnson, published by Little, Brown and Co., Boston.

The quotation on page 59 is from *The Day They Parachuted Cats on Borneo* by Charlotte Pomerantz, © 1971 by Charlotte Pomerantz, published by Addison-Wesley Publishing Company, Reading, Mass. Reprinted by permission.

The quotation on page 69 is from *Hour of Gold, Hour of Lead* by Anne Morrow Lindbergh, published by Harcourt Brace Jovanovich, Inc., New York.

Published by TIMES BOOKS, a division of
The New York Times Book Co., Inc.
Three Park Avenue, New York, N.Y. 10016

Published simultaneously in Canada by
Fitzhenry & Whiteside, Ltd., Toronto

Library of Congress Cataloging in Publication Data

Rossi, Nancy, 1949–
    From this day forward.

    1. Rossi, John F.   2. Cancer—Patients—United
States—Biography.   I. Title.
RC265.6.R67R67   1983   362.1'96994'00924   [B]   83-45040
ISBN 0-8129-1081-8

Designed by Doris Borowsky

Manufactured in the United States of America

83 84 85 86 87 5 4 3 2 1

For John

FROM
THIS DAY
FORWARD

PROLOGUE

There is still some steam on the dining-room windows from the cooking in the kitchen and from the warmth of a room filled with people, as it was an hour ago, and in the corner of one window the steam has turned to frost. I'm wrapped up in an old soft cotton nightgown and Viyella robe with navy-blue knee socks on my feet, which are tucked underneath me, as I sit at the cleared-off dining-room table. God, it looks cold outside, I think; in fact, it must be, because here comes a young man with his head bent down into his neck and chest fighting the winds as he walks up the hill between 86th and 87th streets. He's the only person I can see all up and down Madison Avenue. Even the lighted phone booth across the street looks as if it would rip the skin off your hand if you touched its frozen steel frame. I look down at a pile of seed catalogues in front of me; I've been wanting to look through them since they came a couple of weeks ago, but I was too busy organizing my son's second-birthday party. I spread them out in front of me and realize I don't have a pen or paper to figure my orders out on, so I get up and walk very quietly back to my room to get them, and as I tiptoe back, I stop and stand motionless outside his door. He's not quite asleep. He's talking to himself in his crib in his just-today-two-year-old voice, and he's reviewing everything that happened at his birthday party. I can hear, "Blow candles, candles, blow candles, blow candles, cake, cake, cake and *ice* cream! Happy birthday, happy birthday you, John birthday, John eat cake! John blow candles!" I go back to the dining room. How can two years have passed by so quickly?

The apartment is remarkably still and uncomfortably silent compared to a few hours ago when the laughs of children and adults filled it. Sitting here this cold January night I want to believe that reading seed catalogues and planning for another spring, for another garden, will make me feel better. But it really doesn't: I miss my husband, who died a little more than two years ago. I can feel a wave of feeling sorry for myself cross over my forehead, and I bite my upper lip, sigh, close my eyes and put my head in my hands. I don't even cry. I shake my head. I open my eyes though, and turn to the first page of the Park's seed catalogue, and the first thing I see is that they've got a new squash, Kuta, "a major breakthrough in squash development in this century!" I'm impressed. It'll probably take over the garden, but I think I'll try it, so I write it down. Do I want to do cucumbers again? Yeah, I know, I know, I can hear my mother say that they, too, take over the garden. I write it down anyway. Along with spaghetti squash, pole beans and seeds for geraniums and impatiens that I'll start here on the windowsill. That will be an experiment. It'll be fun to let John help me plant the seeds in the trays and water them every day.

He looked great this afternoon, no kidding. Dressed in his navy-blue flannel, short, fancy overalls with the red-and-white-striped oxford-cloth shirt underneath and his white knee socks and his red shoes. I wish I had the pictures to look at, right now, but they won't be back from the developer for another week. People say he looks exactly like me, and he does, but he also looks exactly like the baby photographs of his father when he was that age. I think that because John, my husband, is not here, I, and everyone else, forget that his son looks so much like him. The main difference is that my husband when he'd grown up had very dark curly hair; my son has light-brown, almost blond, straight hair. But those baby pictures of my husband show the same kind of hair, same color even. My son and I have the same round faces and the same coloring; my eyes are blue, but not the bright piercing blue that my husband's were, and John has inherited his eyes. I just hope that he doesn't inherit my height. I'm not even five feet tall, and my husband at various times and in various moods would call me Little One, Old Short and Round, or Little Shaver, or just plain Nini, the closest a young child I used to baby-sit for could get to Nancy, and the name stuck, at least within my family. So far John's been at average height or above; I hope it stays that way. It will be nice if he grows as tall as his father, but I have my doubts. One thing is clear, though. He's got his father's enthusiasm and anticipation. He's ready for anything every minute he's awake. What he has is confidence. I don't know how he got it; I think often that it just must have been handed to him through his father's genes, as I am quite shy. Whenever I feel blue, as if I am, and what happened to me is, the most tragic thing on earth, I take a good look at my son. If I were such a failure, if I were the unconfident, non-coping person I sometimes think I am when the gray winter skies roll by, then how could I have raised my son to be the person he is? Looking at him is like giving myself a boost of self-confidence, like getting a nonverbal pep talk, which reminds me of the ones my John used to give me. Sometimes he'd sit me down for half an hour and practically shake me into the realization that I was worthwhile. Those years of infertility really blew the shellac off my cover. Month after month would go by, but, oh, well, I'll get into that later.

What I want to say now is that all of us can have our hearts picked up and smashed against a wall, all of us can lose the people dearest to us, all of us can be faced with unfair, cruel tragedies, tragedies seemingly plucked out of the sky and thrown down to us, and while we go through them it *is* as if no one has ever endured such pain, as if no one has ever lived through such hell and sadness, and it's true. No one ever has. No one can enter your head and live the tragedy you're living through even though a similar experience may have befallen them; I think that's why it got so much on my nerves to hear people say to me, "I understand." How on earth could they? They weren't me. But what they could understand was that there was a long road of grieving, mourning and crawling back to life for me. Because *that* they had been through. And they were alive to prove it. And that's just one of the reasons I look at seed catalogues.

I wonder what John would think of the Kuta squash. I just know that "a breakthrough in squash development" would have set him laughing. After renting group houses with friends in East Hampton for a few years, he and I and my divorced parents pooled our money and bought a house in Bridgehampton. John was so excited about it. During the first spring we owned it, we'd race out there every Friday night, along with my mother usually, to paint the inside, which hadn't seen a fresh coat of paint in decades, to buy furniture and beds and kitchen equipment, and most important to me, at least at that time of year, to see what trees, plants and shrubs had bloomed. When we'd first seen the house the fall before, a tiny brown shingle house with white trim, everything was green with that heavy, tired, used, end-of-summer look, and very overgrown. So this first spring had surprises every weekend. First the snowbells poking up so shyly along the foundation of the house. We waited for crocus but none arrived—we'd have to do something about that in the fall, plant some bulbs—but later to compensate there was the surprise of the huge forsythia bushes, which surely hadn't been pruned for years but on their own had become perfect round bushes, six, seven feet high. Grape hyacinth, daffodils, narcissus, thousands of violets, a huge bed of lilies of the valley. The biggest surprise, joy really, was the grove of trees over the violets, scrubby thin things twenty feet high, which I should have recognized but didn't until their distinctive smooth, symmetrical leaves appeared and the fat buds opened to show that, yes, these were lilacs. After a morning of painting the living room, just standing under them and letting the lilac perfume fall onto my face was more reviving than a cup of coffee. I can see John, with paint on his tennis hat, coming out of the house announcing he's finished the last wall and asking, "What do we have for lunch, Little One?" He has a beer in his hand, and I say I'll fix some sandwiches, but then I ask him where he thinks we should have the vegetable garden. We both look at the sun and then down to the ground, estimating which part of the backyard gets the most sun. John walks around very seriously with his beer can, surveying the possibilities. I love that he takes this decision as seriously as I do. He knows how much gardening means to me, how I've longed for this garden and how I want to teach myself year after year so that by the time we're in our sixties I may know what I'm doing. "I think right over there, Nini, behind the garage. It'll be out of the way and yet there'll be maximum sun, because, if I'm right, the back of the garage faces south."

And once we'd decided that the vegetable garden would be eight by ten feet and had staked it off, he broke the ground so effortlessly, did it in one morning, and the next weekend dug the holes for the posts and put the wire fence in around it. He was so strong. He ran every day, played squash and tennis every week, winter and summer. God, I think now, pulling my robe closer around me in the chilly apartment, John was so strong then. And nine months later he didn't have the strength to press down a button on a portable cassette recorder.

CHAPTER ONE

John and I met at a party that neither of us wanted to go to in Manhasset, Long Island, in April 1972.

I was spending the weekend with my friend Lynn, whom I had met a few weeks earlier (we both worked in the Wall Street area, I at Merrill Lynch). Lynn had mentioned that she and a friend of hers were planning a party for people who were not seriously dating one person and would like to meet others, and would I like to spend the weekend at her parents' house and go to this party with her? Inwardly I wasn't very enthusiastic, but I said sure.

A childhood friend of hers from Manhasset was a lawyer with John at Kelley Drye Clark Carr & Ellis, as it was called then, and he had invited John. John also wasn't very enthusiastic, but he said sure; actually he said yes because he wanted to ride in this friend's Ferrari—that's how they were going to get to the party from the city.

There were probably about thirty people at the party, comfortably talking to each other. I didn't know anyone but Lynn, and because she was co-hosting the evening, she had a lot to do. I was left pretty much to myself. I tried joining the conversation with a group of girls sitting on the living-room couch, but I didn't have much to contribute, and trying to look and sound interested in places and people I'd never been to or met, trying to keep an enthusiastic smile on my face, was starting to make me hold back yawns. Most of the young men were standing around the bar.

Looking back on it, I think I may have looked the prettiest I've ever looked that night. My weight was down to 103, and my long light-brown hair had blond streaks in it. I glanced over to the bar but was too shy to get myself a drink. An hour went by. Somehow I just didn't have the strength to make what would have been a tremendous effort to be the center of somebody's, anybody's, attention. I enjoyed observing, and excusing myself from the girls on the couch, I sat down across the room on a turquoise brocade ottoman in front of a lovely Queen Anne wing chair and lighted a cigarette. I remember admiring the simple and graceful carved moldings around the ceiling of the living room, which reminded me of a house my grandparents once lived in in Scarsdale.

It must have been right after I lowered my head from looking at the moldings that I saw the most handsome, the best-looking, the most beautiful young man I'd ever seen walk into the house. He had on a wild pair of red-white-and-blue summer pants, a white button-down shirt without a tie, and a navy-blue blazer. He was with another fellow who seemed to know everybody, and as he walked into the hallway, he had the biggest grin on his face and was shaking hands with the people to whom his friend introduced him. He didn't stop there to chat with any of them; he kept right on walking into the living room, having by this time left his friend behind. He smiled left and right and, without hesitating an instant, kept walking farther and farther into the room, past the girls on the couch, past the couple standing by the fireplace.

I hadn't taken my eyes off him, but now I glanced down at the white-and-blue oriental rug, with no specific thought in my mind, just a hmmm, I wonder who he is, and in a blink and a breath there were two big feet taking up the space where the blue geometric pattern of the rug stopped and the white background began. I looked up at his face and smiled. Because I was sitting on the low ottoman, it was awkward for him to bend over, so he quickly got down on his knees and said, "Hi, I'm John."

And I smiled and said, "Hi, I'm Nancy."

And he said, "I saw you the moment I walked in. You are the most beautiful girl I have ever seen in my life, and someday I'm going to marry you."

Even if they didn't show it, my eyes were rolling around in my head, and I thought, What *is* this? I didn't think it was funny, but I answered dumbly, "Oh, no," and did my best to restore to my face the smile that had vanished, and even to giggle. Nobody had ever said that I was beautiful before, certainly no stranger, and I thought he was either nuts or we were connected by electric wires. How I'd longed for someone to tell me that. I might be considered cute, but because I'm not even five feet tall, the word "beautiful" had never been used about me. And as for the part about marrying me, it had the effect of making me unable to move my lips, to let any more words out. My mouth was half open with only air coming out.

"Let me get you a drink," said John. "I sure as hell need one. I came out here with a fellow I work with in his Ferrari, and he must have been going at least ninety the whole time. I'm a wreck. I'm going to have some bourbon. What would you like, Nancy?"

Weakly, and not even believing his buoyancy, his ease, his confidence and his obvious humor, I told him that a bourbon would be just fine with me, too. Of course I'd never had bourbon before, but that didn't matter. His friend saw him coming back across the room toward the bar and introduced him to a few other people, and John waved his hand over in my direction and indicated he was going right back there with the drinks. He came back, spilling a little bit on his pants, shaking his head and laughing and saying, "Geez, can't take me anyplace." I laughed at that (I, too, am very good at spilling food and drinks over myself and other people's furniture and rugs).

Three hours passed with John sitting on the floor while I sat on that ottoman, and he proceeded to tell me everything about himself. He had been born and had grown up in Utica, New York. He had a brother and two sisters. His father had his own law firm in Utica. He had gone to Colgate because he hadn't gotten into Harvard, where his father had gone, and even though he had been accepted by Williams, his family had wanted him to stay in New York State. He then had gone to Cornell Law School, and had been living in New York City since December 1970, following six months of basic training in the Army Reserve, and was a lawyer in the tax department of a Park Avenue law firm. He had a roommate, with whom he had gone to law school, who preferred to spend his time with much, much older women and loved the ballet, and he'd even fixed John up with a couple of ballet dancers, which John thought was great, but he said he'd never met such egotistical women, and he didn't think they liked him very much anyway.

At about ten o'clock John got up to go, said he had to

catch the train back to New York as he had to get up at dawn the next morning to go to a Reserve meeting. He was really sorry he had to leave. He waved over his friend with the Ferrari, and together they realized he had about two and half minutes to get to the station and make the train, and as quickly as he'd flown into the room three hours before, he was gone. He didn't even know my last name.

He tracked me down, though. Took him about four weeks, and by that time I'd pretty much forgotten about him. He knew I worked at Merrill Lynch, knew his law-firm friend was a friend of Lynn's, and somehow through her got my last name and called me one day at the office. Would I meet him for dinner? We'd have drinks first in the lobby of the Dorset Hotel.

John was waiting for me when I arrived, and I wasn't even late. He had on the worst-looking suit I'd ever seen. Said he'd sent his measurements to some place in Hong Kong. God, it was awful. And once he'd gotten us our drinks, he again talked about himself, but this time he told me how much he made at his law firm, that he'd just come from buying a $250 suit at Saks Fifth Avenue, that the rent for his apartment was $700, that his father had told him to marry a princess. He was a different person. Where, he asked me, did I think the money came from in the family at whose house we'd met? Was the father of the girl really rich? How was I to know? I was squirming.

We left the bar to go to his favorite restaurant, Nirvana, on the top of a building on Central Park South, and I already disliked him. Why all this emphasis on money? Nirvana was very good, because John knew a lot about Indian food and ordered for us both, but he was mad that we hadn't been seated in the terrace room overlooking the Park, and I was mad because the goddam twanging Indian music had set my nerves bouncing, and I had a very hard time hearing him anyway, and then all of a sudden we were joined by John's boss in the tax department and his wife, who'd also decided to have dinner there that night. John was pretty obnoxious and show-offy with them, too, but they were all busy talking, and at least that meant all I had to do was watch. By the time dessert came, I was looking forward to going home and to never seeing John again.

He brought me home and took me up to my apartment. I was so rude I didn't invite him in but instead opened the door with my keys, got down on my knees to pick up one of my two cats, and brought myself and the cat up to John's face and pretty snottily told him thanks and goodnight. I closed the door and heard him walk down the stairs. I was so unhappy. How could anybody who had been so lovely four weeks earlier turn out to be such a phony, interested only in other people's salaries and their material worth? I certainly had misjudged him.

Another four or six weeks went by, and I kept thinking about our first meeting at the party, and kept thinking I wasn't crazy, that there was something there. So I did something I'd never done before. I called him up and asked him over for dinner. He was delighted, and said he'd come.

I made spaghetti, which probably wasn't a smart choice for a man who'd grown up on exquisite Italian cooking, but he was very complimentary. Thought it was great. Thought I was great. Thought the apartment was great. Thought the cats were unnecessary. Saw the bed in the back bedroom and thought that looked great, too.

We finished the spaghetti and the bottle of wine he'd brought along, and were sitting on a pathetic daybed of a couch I had, with the record player on. He leaned over and kissed me, put his arms around me, kissed me again, and said I *smelled* good, in fact said, "My God, you smell good. You smell just like me!" (Maybe our noses were more sensitive than others', but we developed a private theory over the years that people fall in love with people who smell the same as they do.) And I threw my arms around him and we kissed up to the clouds. Our passions grew, and I saw him eyeing that bedroom again, and I just didn't want it to get that far, and fortunately the record needed changing, so I got up to turn it over, and said what a lovely night it had been and thanked him for coming and reached down and picked up a cat. John said he'd had a wonderful time.

He called me about a week later, the night before I was to leave for a vacation by myself in the Caribbean, the first vacation I'd had since I'd started working at Merrill Lynch two years before, and he took me out for dinner. This time when we returned to my apartment I, too, thought the bed looked great, and it was.

I returned from my week's trip on a Friday. Half an hour after I'd paid the cab from Kennedy Airport to my apartment and had begun to unpack, the phone rang.

"Hi, Nancy. This is John Rossi. Where have you been? I called you all last night and then first thing this morning before I left for the office, and there wasn't any answer."

"I just got home."

"Just now?"

"Yes, just a little while ago."

"But I thought you were coming home yesterday."

"No, today."

"Oh, well, at least you're home. I was worried that maybe something had happened to you. Did you have a good trip? How was the weather?"

"Beautiful. I swam every day and walked up and down the beach picking up the most beautiful shells. There weren't many people there, so that was nice, and the ones I met were very friendly, mostly families, one even from

California—a long way to go for a vacation, huh? And I did some shopping in St. Thomas. In fact, I bought you a present."

"You did? What is it? No, give it to me on the train."

"What train?"

"Oh, yeah, well, would you like to come out to the house in East Hampton for the weekend? I'll pick you up in an hour, and we'll get a cab to Penn Station, okay?"

"Oh, gee, John, how nice. Yeah, sure I'd like to come. Thanks."

"That's great, Nancy. I'll be over later."

"Fine, I'll see you then."

I remember hanging up the phone amazed that John had tried to reach me all those times, and here he was asking me out to the beach house he shared with a group of friends from his office, and it hit me that maybe he really liked me. I had a huge smile on my face for the next hour as I sorted from my suitcases things I'd leave and things I'd take with me. I really didn't have much to take, because there wasn't enough time to do the dirty laundry from the trip. It was kind of funny, I thought, that here was my first weekend with John in this summer house, and any other week I'd have been planning every night after work what clothes I would take, really organizing everything to the last item, probably even packing the suitcase as a run-through the evening before, and instead I was trying to find just a couple of clean T-shirts.

I took a quick shower and got into a red-and-white cotton Marimekko dress, brushed out my long hair, got some sandals on my feet, and before I'd zipped up the suitcase, the doorbell rang. There was John. He said we were really late. He'd looked at the train schedule wrong, and we had to make tracks to get to Penn Station in time. We ran down the stairs out to the street, and John sped ahead up the block to Second Avenue. Miraculously, even as an unexpected shower was beginning to sprinkle fat dots on the sidewalk, an empty cab stopped for him, and we got in.

The driver didn't think we had much of a chance to make a 5:52 train but said he'd do his best, which he certainly did. As he screeched up to Penn Station, John stuffed some dollar bills through the change-box opening, thanked the driver, and we both got out of the cab running. We laughed through the rain, and racing as fast as we could in the sea of the commuter crowd, we eventually reached the long line at the information desk. We looked for a departure board in vain, and John said, "Oh, damn, damn, triple damn." It was now 5:50.

I saw in his face for that instant a look I naively thought men never took on; perhaps a better way to explain it is that I saw an emotion on his face that made me fall permanently in love with him. Stupidly I had thought only women knew what this feeling was like. But I was wrong. Because John, sweat pouring from his face that hot, raining, humid night, standing with his suitcase in one hand, tennis racquet poking out of it, and my suitcase in his other hand, and his gray suit so hot and crumpled, looked as if he were going to cry; he looked as if all his plans, his work for making this a special trip and weekend for us both, were going to fall through. It was so easy to see that while I'd been away on my vacation, he'd spent every night after work during the week planning for this trip. He'd had it all arranged, and now he couldn't even find the damn train. This all happened so fast I didn't even have time to tell him not to worry, that we could wait and get the next train, because he quickly brightened his eyes and put on a smile and said, "Listen, I think Bruce told me they always leave from track eighteen. Let's make a run for it, and maybe we'll be lucky."

So off we went again, dodging closed but dripping umbrellas dangling from people's arms and trying to run as carefully as we could on the wet floor. We finally saw Track 18, which, thinking back on it, must have been, in that cavern, at least three or four city blocks away from where we started, and it did say Montauk! The metal gate was just about to be pulled across by a conductor, but he looked around and saw John waving a suitcase over his head and yelling, "Hold it," and he let us through. We ran down the ramp onto the first car and stood next to a couple holding a baby. We heard the doors slide closed behind us and felt the train begin to move out. We had made it. John was so relieved. Now the weekend could go forward; it hadn't been ruined.

We changed trains at Jamaica station and were lucky to get a couple of seats together right behind that same young couple with the baby. John bought us a couple of beers, and while he drank his, he played peek-a-boo and made funny faces at the baby, who was being held against his father's shoulder, allowing him to peer over the seat and look at us. John made the baby laugh and laugh until the little boy was tired enough to sleep on his parents' laps. The rest of the way out we talked, and John reminded me about his present, which I gave him right away. It was a Liberty-print tie I'd bought in St. Thomas. He told me I had excellent taste in ties. I am not modest; I do.

The air conditioning in the train never really worked during the whole three-hour ride, so when we got off at the East Hampton station, the cool night air was a wonderful surprise. It had been an unusually hot early-June day in the city, but out here it was almost cold, and we both shivered. John got one of the cabs in the station parking lot to take us to the house, which was right in the village. The cab pulled into the driveway of a big Spanish-style stucco house with red tile roof and green shutters at the windows and even a fancy black grillwork wrought-iron balcony above the massive wooden front door. We were the first to arrive, it seemed, for the house was dark.

John paid the driver and proceeded to figure out which of the dozen keys in his key case belonged to the house. He'd had it made during the week, but in the dark he couldn't tell which was the shiny new one, so he tried them all. It was so peaceful standing under the doorway. The trees that arched over the street were quietly dripping the excess rain off their leaves onto the road. It made a nice noise. The lawn all around the house must have been mowed that afternoon before it had started to rain, because the fresh green smell was still strong.

The next key John put into the lock turned easily, and the door opened. He flipped the outdoor and then the hall lights on, and we walked into the dark house. The first thing we wanted to do, we agreed, was change out of our sweaty, now clammy and cold, clothes. He got into some jeans and a clean faded madras shirt, and I pulled out an old pair of white Army/Navy-store pants and an old Brooks pink oxford-cloth shirt and put on a long-sleeved navy-blue-and-white sun-print T-shirt on top of it.

We were both a little awkward, now having finally arrived, and we went down to the kitchen to see if there was anything to eat and to get something to drink, and while John made us each a gin and tonic, he began to talk a mile a minute about the house, his work, anything to fill up the silence of the house. I decided to lift myself up to sit on the countertop, thinking I would look neat sitting up there listening to him as he made our drinks. Because I am short, this was a hard maneuver in any kitchen, but this house seemed to have even higher than usual countertops. I put my hands and arms out behind me and reached up so that they were touching the countertop; then I quickly placed my hands palms down and with great energy and agility, quietly and really skillfully, lifted myself up over the coun-

ter. John turned and looked at me admiringly. Gee, for
such a little thing, she's awfully strong, I could hear him
thinking. I was still in midair, my backside just about to
touch down on the counter; I was smiling with such self-
satisfied pride on my face, the same way I used to when I
was a trampoline champion at my grade school, and I was
smiling because I could feel John's approval and also because I knew I was showing off. John turned back to his
drink-fixing, and I landed, not as quietly as I'd hoped, in a
plate, yes, in a dinner plate full of the previous weekend's
accumulated bacon grease, which because of the warm
weather hadn't solidified except for the merest crust of fat
across the top.

Aw shit, I thought. My attempt at elegance and sophis-
tication in the Hamptons. I couldn't imagine what the reaction from John was going to be, because I didn't know
him that well yet.

I said, "John," and he replied, "Yes, Nancy," and
turned his head toward me. "Look what I've done." I
gulped, let out a long breath quietly to give me courage
and said, "I'm sitting in bacon grease." My left hand
instinctively went up to my face to cover half of it in
embarrassment, and what could be seen of my eyebrows
were wrinkled questioningly toward John, with my eyes
peering out underneath them, and I started to giggle
nervously.

"Oh, my God, Nancy. Oh, I'm sorry. Boy, who would
have left bacon fat in a goddam plate?" And then I heard
a groan from him. "Uh, Nancy, I remember." And he
stretched his face into a forced but scared smile. "Uh, I
was supposed to have cleaned up that plate before we left
last Sunday, and I guess when the maid was here this
week, she thought we'd left it there for a purpose. I am
really sorry. Here let me help you down. Oh, gee, you are
really covered in it, your pants are ruined, I think. Oh,
dear, oh, dear."

"It's all right," I said. "I can't believe how stupid I am. I'll go up and change."

But John poked his face up into mine and smiled up at me with his lips pressed together. His eyes were dancing, and he began to laugh and threw his arms around me, hugged me, and lifted me off the kitchen countertop, and hugged me again so tightly to him, put his face into the side of my neck, and said, "You are fantastic."

He grabbed my hand and pulled me with him, flying, around the corner, through the still-dark living room, past his briefcase still left on the floor, and up the stairs, stopping briefly to turn on a light, and then still running, down the hall, back through the door of his bedroom. He flopped backward onto the double bed and pulled me down on top of him. We were both laughing so hard. "Jesus, Nancy," he said, "let's get these pants off!"

And before anyone else had arrived at the house, we'd made love in his bed, gotten dressed again, with my white pants a wadded, greasy ball left on the closet floor, run back downstairs and cleaned up the bacon-grease plate. We were elegantly having our gin and tonics when the others arrived. Years later John would say, "Oh, you should have seen yourself sit in the bacon grease. I couldn't believe you were a native New Yorker, because all the New York City women I'd met were so perfect, and you were so normal. If I hadn't been in love with you before, I sure was then!"

But for the next year and half we had a grueling courtship. Lots of fun and lots of fights. We'd see each other every night and day for weeks, and then we wouldn't talk to each other for a month or more. We must have had a surplus of emotional energy to stand it, but we persevered, and in time we were married, though I guess I would have to admit that I was the one who finally asked him.

We began living together in a small one-bedroom apart-

ment a year and a half after that first summer, an apartment we rented together, and we'd been in there about six
months when one day I joked with him and said we were
going to go downtown that Saturday morning to look at
engagement rings.

"Really, Nini?" he said. "Do we have to?"

"Yes, John, we have to," I replied.

So we went to Cartier's, where my father had had my
mother's engagement ring made, and John and I looked
around in an equally stunned silence. "Well, Nini, what
do you like?"

Gulping, I replied that I'd always liked sapphires, that I
didn't want a diamond ring, and besides they were way
too expensive, and we couldn't afford it. John then took
over and got a salesman to help us. This icy older man
with a balding head and carefully enunciated words very
soon started to smile and talk and laugh with John. They
weren't even talking about rings. John was doing what he
always did, asking the man how long he'd worked there,
how much training went into being an expert about all
these different stones, and whether he liked his work, and
when the subject finally turned to rings and families, the
man told us about his daughter and son-in-law who'd just
gotten married, and instead of intimidating us, the man
couldn't have been nicer. He showed us every sapphire
ring he had for the amount we felt we could spend. He
didn't even suggest more expensive rings.

John saw one in the case, though, that he particularly
liked and asked me if I liked it. We could tell the man liked
it, because he smiled and nodded at John approvingly,
and he quickly put it on the velvet tray with the others,
and I leaned over the counter to get a better look at it. I
couldn't believe it. It was perfect. It fulfilled every romantic notion I'd ever had. A sapphire ring with a couple of
small pear-shaped diamonds all set in shining gold. As

John helped me to try it on, I remember looking at the still, peaceful navy color of that sapphire and thinking that focusing on that blue water-like stone would help me whenever I got nervous.

John looked at me. Did I really like it? Oh, yes, and I squeezed his hand. The man told us we could pick it up in a few weeks after it had been made the right size for me. John then opened a charge account, and it was done.

We thanked that kind man and walked out into what had turned into a snowstorm, not a windy one, but just a steady fall of billowing flakes. It must have been not much below freezing, because it felt warm, and without even thinking about it, we walked up Fifth Avenue past the stores, without looking at them, and past the fountain in front of the Plaza, and finally walked on the sidewalk alongside the park. All we did was talk, not so much about what we'd just done but about each other and how happy we were.

One thing John and I could do was talk, talk, talk. They were rarely the most profound conversations in the world, but we had a running dialogue each day, and John would even call me at my office two or three times a day just to chat, and when we went to bed at night, we might both have had the sure intention of reading a book or reading papers for work as we lay back on the pillows against the headboard, but after only five or ten minutes, we'd start to talk. What did John think about this; what did I think about that? Guess who I saw today? Did you read Bernard Gwertzman's latest report about Watergate? Where do you want to go to dinner Friday night? Wasn't it nice that spring training had started? Well, of course, the Yankees'll have a good year. I'll stick to the Mets, thanks, John, all American League players still remind me of Boog Powell. You know who Boog Powell was? Sure, John. First base Baltimore. Wait a minute, I think I can remember their entire 1969 lineup. No you can't. Sure I can. Oh, but Nini, you'd have to have grown up in Utica, listening to the games on the radio on hot summer days, to know what it was like to love the Yankees back then. Hey, Nini, you're not going to read, are you? No. Good, let's um ah, you know what I mean. Oh, yes, um ah, I know what you mean. And we'd wink at each other devilishly and throw the covers over our heads and giggle. And even afterward, as we were dozing off, we'd still be whispering to each other in the dark, just like a couple of children.

By the zoo, where John would get his tennis permit every spring, the snow was sticking to the ground and covering the black March branches above us. "Do you want to get a bus, Nini?" he asked. "Oh, no, let's walk the rest of the way home." The snow continued to fall all afternoon and evening. We turned on the afternoon opera broadcast, and while I started cutting up vegetables for a big pot of soup I was going to make that night, John started baking a loaf of bread—well, really, one big loaf and one very little loaf. I'd given him James Beard's bread cookbook for Christmas. John had said a few times that he'd like to learn, and since Christmas, he'd made bread almost every weekend, and we'd both gained a few pounds. John had gotten out of his nice going-downtown-to-look-at-engagement-rings clothes, and I was out of my light-blue polka-dot silk dress that John had gotten me for Christmas, and we both put on some corduroy pants and turtlenecks that had been through the washing machine with the bleach in it and now had splotches all over them.

We ate our soup-and-bread supper with a few glasses of red jug wine, and after watching *Star Trek* and *Kojak* John turned to me and said, "You really want to get married, don't you?" I nodded my head quietly without lifting my eyes up to look at him, and he said, "You know, Nini, I will never get a divorce. If we get married, that's it. *Capisce?*"

I looked at him. I realized then how seriously he took the subject. He didn't want any part of it if either of us thought in the back of our minds, Oh, hell, if it doesn't work out, we can get a divorce. I hadn't taken the idea, the state of marriage as seriously as he did, and he knew it. "I understand," I finally said.

Then he turned off the television by extending his leg and pushing in the off button with his foot, and very seriously he took my hands in his and asked me to marry him, to be his wife. I can feel even now how my eyes became wet inside, and blinking a lot, I answered yes. John then jumped up, still holding my hands, and pulled me up with him. "Great, it's settled," he said.

"You're sure you want to do this, John?"

"Oh, Nini, of course. Come on, get your boots on, and let's go get the paper."

We always bought the Sunday paper late Saturday night so we wouldn't have to get dressed first thing Sunday morning, and John usually did this errand alone, but tonight we could see, although just barely, that outside our apartment, with no view of anything except brick walls, the snow was still falling and was deep on the ground. We put on our hats, coats, scarves and gloves, and when we opened the door of the building and walked out onto the sidewalk, all we could hear was the whooshing sound of the snow blowing down.

It was eerie. There were no fresh tire tracks on the street; even the 67th Street crosstown bus, which went past our building, obviously hadn't been along in a while. In fact, we couldn't even hear the buses on Third Avenue in one direction and on Second in the other. Just the whooshing, blowing snow in the midst of great stillness. It was so strange that instead of going right to the newsstand on the corner, we walked aimlessly, randomly, looking at familiar objects and sights in an unfamiliar cover of six inches of white, not yet dirty snow. We walked around the neighborhood seeing the sharp angles of the city turn softer, rounder. The 90-degree angle of a building at a corner lost its jab with a drift of snow up against it.

Everything looked friendly but secretive. On the south side of an apartment building on 66th Street, we peered through the fence railing and saw the building's interior garden sparkling with snow, with the lights from the restaurant that looked out on it still giving a fairyland glow to the snow-covered trees and shrubs. We looked down at our feet and saw that ours were the first footprints to be made here. Right outside that garden the snow was so untouched and perfect that although we didn't say it, neither of us wanted to disturb it. It wasn't until we walked a little bit farther and saw that other prints had been made in the snow and that snow had been grabbed off cars to make snowballs that we felt comfortable enough to do the same. John was the first to scoop up a handful of snow, and then I did, and then we started to throw handful after handful of snow into the air. The snow was too light and dry to be packed into good snowballs, so we just kept throwing the snow high above our heads like confetti, but under the light of the streetlamp it came down to us looking more like magic twinkling fairy dust. We held back our heads and turned our faces skyward so that we could look at this miracle snow falling back onto our faces and melting there.

I think now how wonderful it would be to create the same swirling, sparkling, icy-cold snow effect at the beginning of the third act of *La Bohème*. The snow in a stage production always comes down so vertically, sometimes lighter or heavier in its density but really never changing direction. At least that's the way I remember it the night John announced our engagement to our closest friends at a performance of *La Bohème*.

New, fresh, falling snow under a New York City street-lamp may be one kind of fairyland, nature's fairyland, but the Opera Club is another, a man-made fairyland. Of course, I was in love with one of the handsomest young men in the world, and he made me feel like one of the prettiest women who had ever lived, so my eyes may have been clouded by love and romance and the general goodness of life at the time, but I will always remember the room of the Opera Club as one of the most exquisitely beautiful rooms in the world. It made every man look handsome and every woman look as if fairy godmothers were still alive to find beautiful dresses and to give each face a welcoming joyous smile. It sounds antiquated. It was and it is, I suppose, but anyone who has ever been there is made to feel like royalty, and once treated to this, in person instead of just hearing about it, has never sneered. Yes, it is a men's club. Yes, no women are allowed to be members. Yes, as a widow I cannot now be a member. Strangely, that does not bother me. I am, I know, dumb about these things.

I loved reading *Time and Again*, about a young man in the 1970s who agrees to participate in a government research project, which instead of looking into the future looks into the past. The government rents an apartment in the Dakota, and he looks out the window one snowy evening, sees the taxis going up and down Central Park West, and the next moment he's seeing horsedrawn sleighs instead. I know, Jacob Riis, those soul-shattering pictures of the squalor and poverty at the time, I know all that, but once, letting our romantic fancies fly, wouldn't it be nice to ride in a horsedrawn sleigh in your fur hat and fur muff next to a man in a top hat with a laprobe over both of you on your way to the opera in the 1880s? Maybe dinner at Sherry's first? Do you know anyone who would turn that down?

Well, an evening at the Opera Club in 1974 was as close
to that as anything I've experienced except perhaps skat-
ing on a frozen winter pond at night or a summer party on
the lawn in front of a rambling nineteenth-century summer house, both in East Hampton. I'd had my own subscription to the opera before I'd even met John, but it was
only after John began taking me to the Opera Club that I
realized it was there. We would enter it at intermission
and leave it when the chimes rang to return to our seats;
before I always must have passed it when the doors were
closed.

On that special night, John seemed anxious to get to the
opera house. "Oh, Little One," he said impatiently from
the bedroom, "get out of there. Come on, let's go." I came
out of the bathroom, looked at John and saw him still
struggling with the studs in his shirt. As usual, I was
dressed before he was, but he liked to tease me and pretend that I was the stereotypical always-late woman. I
looked at him now with my hands on my hips, and saw
that aside from the formal shirt into which he was vainly
trying to place the studs, the only other items he had on
were his shorts and his black silk socks held up by garters.
He looked so incredibly handsome: his hair was still a little
wet and curling from his shower, and though he hated
shaving twice in one day, he had done it to please me. I
put the studs in for him, as I would do countless times
during the next years, during our marriage, and I realize
now that that was one of the sweetest moments of our life
together, one that I miss so much now—the times he
would lift his chin up, and I'd put those studs in his formal
shirt. Then he put on his grandfather's gold cufflinks, ini-
tialed GR (his grandfather, although called John by his
medical colleagues in Utica, was born in Italy as Giovanni
Rossi). The worst part was the black tie, and neither of us
knew how to tie one very well; one side always shot up

under his chin. When it was done, John flew into the rest of his clothes, and we were off.

We took the 67th Street crosstown bus over to Lincoln Center. We got off at Broadway, and my feet in evening shoes, which didn't really fit me, took small fast steps to keep up with John. As we walked across the plaza, past the fountains toward the Chagall murals whose colors looked particularly bright that crackling cold evening, my long black evening coat flapped around me in the wind, showing the light-blue satin dress underneath, and my hair and John's flew around our faces.

He stopped as we reached the glass cases displaying the casts of the week's coming performances and lightly touched my shoulder and said, "Nini, don't mention to anyone that we're going to get married, all right?"

"Well, okay," I said slowly, "but why not?"

"Let's just wait awhile, wait until the ring comes, maybe."

"All right, Bunky, if that's what you want, I won't tell anybody." And I forgot it.

Then I asked him, as I would every opera night in our future, "Can I buy a libretto, Bunky?" I loved asking him this question, because each time—even years later when our finances could absorb lots of librettos—he pretended he was angry and told me that it was such an extravagance, how would we ever have money saved for anything if I kept buying librettos?

"Oh, come on, Bunky, please?"

"Oh, all right," he answered, "but this is the last one." He winked and said, "I mean it."

Then he opened the door for us, the only one that is unlocked at that early hour, the one by the ticket booths, and waited for me there while I ran to the ticket takers and ushers hanging around the bottom of the Grand Staircase to see if one of them would sell me one of the librettos piled on a nearby table. One of them did, even though the older man who regularly sold them wasn't there yet. Then I paid him with a couple of dollars—John was right, it really was an extravagance; doing that meant I probably wouldn't have enough money to pick up the laundry the next day—and I raced back with the libretto under my arm, and we walked back to the elevator near the gift and souvenir desk.

We could feel we were the center of everyone's attention as we walked back. The lobby was quite full with people buying tickets, selling tickets, with people arriving to eat at the Opera Café down below and with people just sitting on the low windowsills, waiting for a friend to show up. We were the only ones so dressed up. We were young and attractive and happy and in love, and people were looking at our shining eyes, at our confidence in life and the goodness it surely held for us. Certainly, I thought no other young couple had ever felt the way we did, and that must have showed on my face, because elderly women and men particularly returned our stardust gaze with sweet comprehending looks of their own.

We pushed for the elevator, and when it came we rode up and the doors opened directly in the club. And that is where the fairy tale really began. Beyond the small coatroom area by the elevator, the room expanded to a dark, romantic, twinkling dining room. It reminded me of being on an ocean liner, as if we were in the jewel-like dining room of a ship in the middle of a black night sea. The walls were dark, and the tall narrow windows across the room looked out onto the dark night and the Henry Moore sculpture and pool. There were mirrors and trimmings of brass and gold and candles and bright white tablecloths. The crystal chandeliers and the glasses on the table shone off one another, the silverware gleamed. The lighting was soft yet not annoyingly dark, and it was easy to greet recognized faces as we made our way to our table. David Clark and his wife, Carolyn, and Rodd Reynolds and his girlfriend, Janet Tracy, were already there. We sat down and ordered Manhattans for ourselves, and soon we saw our guests, John's boss, Bill Rubinstein, and Sheryl, his wife—the same couple who had been with us at Nirvana—arrive, and waved so that they saw us. It was a crowded evening, and the eight of us were at a table next to one of the windows in the back of the room. David asked for the wine list and asked the waiter what the dinner was that night. A couple of bottles were ordered.

During dinner we talked about the day just ended, our jobs, and the fact that in a little over two months the rental would start on the big house we shared on Georgica Pond in East Hampton and how much we were looking forward to getting out there again. John and David thought maybe they would buy a Sunfish together to sail on the pond. I smiled to myself. Janet told us some opera gossip that she had heard from her voice teacher and also told us that Pavarotti kisses any woman who comes backstage to meet him. We tried to imagine what that would be like and teased the men at the table that maybe the women of this group would give it a try. With that the chimes were played, and we knew it was time to get to our seats. Libretto and opera glasses in hand, I followed John out of the club and up the stairs to our box. As we opened the door, the Austrian snowflake crystal chandeliers were just passing our eyes on their way up to the ceiling, their progress coinciding with the dimming of the lights. We settled into our chairs, the conductor appeared, and the music began. I thought how lucky I was to be sitting there about to hear this opera but most important to be sitting next to John, knowing that he and I would be married, and I reached to squeeze his hand. And in the dark I could see his lips move to say I love you.

The first act was over quickly, Pavarotti at once frolicking with his roommates in the garret and also tenderly, profoundly holding Mimi's cold hand. The opera is so overloaded with sentiment, so overly melodramatic, that I wondered sitting there why I loved it so much and loved all operas with, for the most part, their ridiculous books. In fact, the silly story lines had always given me comfort and reassurance because the lives being sung about, I thought, were so much more theatrically tragic than mine could ever be. I looked back at John and saw the incredible contrast between what was happening on stage and what our lives held for us. We were young, untouched by great sadness, and were therefore able to look at the plot with great tolerance and even appreciation as an exaggerated flight into sentiment. It was a fine way to spend an evening, and it was an escape, but who did we know who might wind up dying like Mimi? No one. So we accepted the story itself as nonsense, but nonsense with a purpose, as it allowed the singers to express life's raw emotions through music, and every emotion at that, all in the span of one evening. We clapped wildly as Scotto and Pavarotti took their first-act bows. The joyous Café Momus second act must have done something to John, though, because as we went back to the club for the intermission the first thing he did was tell everyone that he and I were going to be married, that he had asked me and I'd said yes, that we were engaged. The words spilled out of him and he couldn't stop them, and then he looked so happy and pleased.

David and Rodd leaped to their feet to get the attention of the maître d'. Yes, a bottle of champagne here for this table. Yes, very happy news here. Well, congratulations, Mr. Rossi. The waiters flurried to get the tulip champagne glasses on the table. Everyone toasted us, and others in the room turned their heads to see what was going on. They could tell it was something very good indeed.

The fights and high-voltage behavior of our courtship were behind us, and to our amazement we never had a serious, cruel fight after the day of our wedding. Even the question of religion wasn't a problem; although I had been baptized in the Episcopal church and John was Catholic, we both knew how much it would mean to his parents to be married in a Catholic church. So we were. Our marriage relaxed us, and we flew back and forth, and most often concurrently, as two summer seagulls at dusk flying over the summer beach in East Hampton. We had friends, we both enjoyed our work, we spent what money we had extravagantly on each other, and we talked together for hours and hours at a time. Perhaps the best example of how much we loved each other is that whenever we passed an older, gray-haired couple as we walked along the beach in summer, John would give me a squeeze, and I'd give him a hug, and I'd look up into his dark-blue eyes, and he'd look down to my pale blue eyes, and we'd smile and smile, and we'd finally express it in words: we looked forward to the time when *we'd* be the gray-haired couple walking down the beach, with our lifetime of accomplishments and children and grandchildren behind us, and still in love with each other. John used to say, "You'll be so beautiful then, Nini. I can see you with your gray hair coming out from underneath one of your crazy beach hats or scarves that you'll still be wearing." And I remember telling John that his gray hair would make him look like a Supreme Court judge, that his jokes would be just as funny, and that he'd still be so sexy that I'd still be after him.

It didn't turn out that way.

CHAPTER TWO

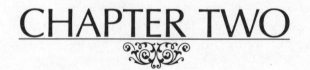

J ohn, can you hear me? Yeah, over here, in the garden.
Listen, would you bring me the Park's seed box on the
porch? Thanks."

"Here, Nini." He looked up at the sky. It was the
spring of 1978. "You don't think it's too cold to plant?"

"No, but I'm just planting the radishes, peas and lettuce.
They're supposed to go in in April or even March. What are
you up to?"

"I'm just about finished with the living room, but I
thought I'd get some coffee, come out here and watch
you. What are you going to do first?"

"Well, I thought I'd do the radishes in this first row.
They don't last that long, and later I can plant something
else in their space. Then I thought a row of peas and then
some lettuce. What d'you think?"

"Sounds good to me. I'm going to get my coffee, Nini. Want anything?"

"No thanks, Bunk." And I went back to placing the radish seeds in the row, covering them as I went along, as I'd read you were supposed to do. John came out and sat on the ground drinking his coffee. It was a warm early-April day, and both of us were in shirtsleeves. The sun gave its first indication on our faces and backs of the warmth it had waiting for us in summer. The golden warmth went right to our winter bones and felt so good. John lay down on his back with his face right into the sun and closed his eyes. We'd been married three and a half years. Gosh, I thought, though, this would be our seventh summer together coming up. We'd been through a lot so far, and I looked over at John, who looked so relaxed lying on the grass, and loved this new house so much, and I kept saying to myself in my head, I just adore this man. God, he always made me laugh.

I finished putting in the radish seeds and then the peas and lettuce. John opened his eyes, and I told him I had finished. It just needed to be watered. Oh, no, we both realized at the same time, we didn't have a hose yet. John jumped up and laughed. He would water it, he said, with the big watering can in the garage.

This I had to see. I even got out my mother's camera and took a picture of him doing it. It took him at least fifty trips back and forth from the outdoor faucet to cover the area. Even Leo, our Burmese cat, moved his head from side to side watching John make all those trips. We crossed our fingers and hoped it would rain during the week.

It was almost noon, and we realized that we had to hurry. Have lunch, clean up the paint trays and brushes, lock up the house, and get on our way back to New York, because we had a late-afternoon appointment with Dr. Uscher over in his New Jersey office. He was the doctor who had been treating our infertility problems, and that day I was to have my usual twice-weekly, soon-to-be-daily, exam. It had been two and a half years since our first pregnancy, which was a tubal pregnancy. What a night that had been. And now after that, and after surgery to open up the remaining fallopian tube, we were on the road of hormones, most likely. We had been charting our sex life on a temperature chart for a couple of years, and we had even given up at one point, started seeing social workers about adopting a child, and then gone back to Dr. Uscher. John would be going to Europe next month, so we knew that this month, April, had to be it. So our visits to Dr. Uscher would occur daily soon, but first we had to get back for that afternoon's appointment.

As John packed the car, I made a mad dash around the house to find the cat. He actually liked traveling in the car, but he just wanted to make finding him hard for us. At last he gave himself away by meowing and running out of the bushes. But then John remembered he wanted to bring back some of his tennis racquets because he had a couple of games that week. One racquet wasn't good enough; he brought three.

At last we were all in the car, and John started the engine. We got onto the Montauk highway, and by the time we reached the Shinnecock Canal we might as well have been in New York. That was the end of Long Island to me, and the rest of the drive was just to be endured. It frightened me a bit, because I'd never learned how to drive. No, that's not accurate. I'd had lessons off and on since I was eighteen, but I had failed one road test in New York and another in Colorado when I was in college. The examiner in Colorado even said I should *never* be allowed to drive I was so rotten. I failed that test because I didn't know what the sign "Soft Shoulders" meant, and slid the car off the road; I failed the New York test because I forgot to take off the emergency brake. So John would turn on the radio, and I would tune out for the rest of the trip. Going home just wasn't as much fun as driving out. And the best weekend to drive out was Memorial Day weekend, the first weekend of summer. It always reminded me of the summer before our marriage when we drove out to Bayberries, that house on Georgica Pond.

Bayberries is a late-nineteenth-century house in East Hampton. It had been built for and owned by the successive generations of one family. It was to be lived in only in summers, for there was no basement for insulation, and fireplaces in the living room, dining room, and two of the bedrooms provided the only heat on cold nights until a gas heater was installed in the living room. The kitchen still had its original wood cooking stove with a pipe going into its own flue. Images of servants wearing caps, holding their long hair up above their hot necks on a summer day, and wearing their white floor-length aprons; of young children in white, with their nurse and mother in high-necked white lawn dresses, waving to Daddy and his friends in their white plus-fours, shirts and caps, as they walked up the porch steps, hot after completing a morning's golf game, eyeing with smiles of relief the pitcher of iced tea or lemonade Mother was pouring into glasses just for them—all these people were still alive when one walked up the lawn from the pond on a hot, bright-blue summer morning. The house had never died.

The first time my husband and I saw the house was on a gray, rainy day in February 1973. We and our friends David and Carolyn Clark had seen many houses that morning with the real estate agent. We were looking for a large house to accommodate us and some other friends for the summer. We were an offshoot from a group house of the previous summer. How could we know that gray day that this house would work its way into our lives and become as permanent and as treasured as an old friend? As we walked through the cold, dark, damp house, which had been locked up all winter, the furniture covered with old white cotton sheets, mentally arranging ourselves in each room—oh *this* is our bedroom—we were sure this was the house for us for the summer.

"Oh, it's so expensive."

"But a good deal for the space—seven bedrooms!"

"And the little beach on the pond."

"The view of the ocean."

"I don't know, though—it's an awful lot."

"Old, too—do you think the others will like it?"

"Needs painting."

"At least the kitchen has a dishwasher."

"And the owners said they'd put in a clothes washer and dryer."

"We'd have to have that."

"But it's beautiful."

"Don't you love the old light fixtures?"

"And the fringed shawl over the piano!"

"A piano for Janet!"

"But there aren't any showers!"

"Those funny cast-iron tubs."

"We can put up shower heads."

"There's plenty of space for a garden."

"I can grow my herbs!"

"Do you think we can find enough people to pay for it?"

"Let's take it."

As it turned out, I wasn't in the house too often that summer. John and I were in the worst time of our three-year courtship, and during the summer of 1973 we hated each other's guts. He still wanted to date a former girl-friend, sleep with her as well as with me. He thought it made sense, was a pretty classy arrangement; I thought it stank. Actually, nobody seemed to fit into that first group living in the house that summer: a little bit too much of "Hey, John, you ate all *my* bacon" and "I asked for a cheeseburger, not a fish sandwich!" But by the summer of 1974, John and I had been living together for six months, David had found others to join the house to take the places of those who'd decided to go off on their own, and more to the point for me and John, we were going to be married in September. The group that eventually assembled in the house that summer were people to whom any one of us would now fly to be of assistance, even to care for our collective brood of children.

And for the next two summers this is how Memorial Day weekend started: that Friday summer evening, John and I were the first to arrive. Even in the dark the house was friendly. John got out his key, opened the door, turned on the porch light and went in to turn on a couple of lamps. I followed with a couple of suitcases and that craning, peering-neck feeling, "Well, this is it, here we are!" We saw so many things we hadn't remembered. And, this time of year was the season the house awoke to. Yes, the cleaning woman had been there: the sheets were off the funny old furniture, bedspreads were on the beds, at the windows were white curtains that would billow all summer in the breeze and lie flat as oilcloth on hot airless days, area rugs were on the floors in the bedrooms. The refrigerator was working. Just then Carolyn and David drove up in the darkness, and they had the same wide-eyed, happy joy of entering this home for the first time since last October. Carolyn and I got our sheets out from our suitcases to make our beds. She and David were in the yellow room, John and I in the pink room—both rooms fronting the lawn, pond and ocean. David and John opened beers and tried to remember how the gas heater in the living room worked while Carolyn and I continued our homemaking tasks, making our bedrooms ours. We fin-

ished, put some food away in the kitchen, and opened
some beers for ourselves. How about a fire? Sure! David
got logs from the back porch, which he had ordered delivered over the spring, and he and John began their home-
steading and sheltering work. The division of labor may
have seemed extraordinarily traditional, but the next days
saw John vacuuming and doing laundry and David sew-
ing up a torn curtain in the living room and setting the
table while other men in the house, for instance David
Barry and Peter and Rodd, baked pies, basted roast ca-
pons and made poached fish with mousseline sauce while
the women were out on the tennis court!

And here was a typical Saturday night in July and August: I was sitting in one of the old wooden deck chairs
from a ship out on the porch at about seven o'clock. I had
showered and washed and dried my hair and dressed for
the evening. A long summer day full of trying to pretend I
could play tennis, trying to pretend I could make John
proud of me, although playing tennis was agony for me. I
hated being watched by others. I was so awful. No hand-
eye coordination. Then beautiful, lazy hours at the beach,
swimming, talking on our towels, drinking beer, everyone
laughing. I was all right then. But the dinners in the evening were my time. Helping with dinner, watching John
tell his stories at the dinner table, that was my time. I
shined. But first, outside alone, while the others were
showering after more early-evening tennis, with a vodka
and tonic.

I was in a long cotton dress, my glass was making water
rings on the arm of the wooden chair because of the foggy
humidity. A cigarette. The lime in my glass was coming to
the top. I looked out across the lawn and saw that the fog
was coming closer to the house off the ocean and the
pond. Everything smelled so good. There was a breeze,
but it was still warm enough for me to be outside with-

out a sweater. I looked at thousands of bugs around the porch lamp. Ugh. "Oh, hi, Hal. Yes, hasn't it been a beautiful day?" The Carly Simon *Hotcakes* album was on the record player in the living room, and I could hear it clearly through the open windows. The song "Safe and Sound"—that was John and me. We would always be safe and sound. The breeze was blowing gently. It was the most wonderful of nights. Here came Teri. Oh, she looked so pretty. "Do you have a cigarette?" Sure. Now there were three of us out on the porch. I almost wanted it to stay this way. Just a few of us out here on the porch, enjoying this special end of the day with the fog over the lawn. No activity. But then, oh, yes, dinner. "I'll go get the cheese and crackers." Oh, the wonderful cheese Carolyn brought out from Zabar's. . .

Port-wine cheese will bring back those summers in an instant. How has any group of people ever been so happy? So secure? A couple of years later we were to learn of Hal and Civi's separation and divorce.

"Nancy, I was always so jealous of you at Bayberries," Civi would say to me.

"Of me?" Me, who was a klutzy tennis player, always overweight compared to the other women, jealous of me?

"Yes. John, the way he looked at you. He adores you. Everyone could see it."

"Adores me? Me?"

"Oh, Nancy, don't you know that?"

And I really hadn't. I had known he loved me, that he was happy, but adored me? Now I realized that, yes, it was true. Oh, how much I had to be grateful for.

To get back to those journeys out of the city each Memorial Day weekend, we'd drive out around seven on the Friday evening of the weekend, hoping to miss most of the traffic, which we did. The car was filled with all our summer clothes, sheets and towels, and all of John's tennis racquets. Tennis racquets that had been repaired, ones that needed new strings, and one brand-new one. For a person who hated clutter and would throw anything away—bills, checks, along with the newspapers and magazines—in order to get back down to the tops of tables, he was a squirrel about tennis racquets and tennis balls.

He once read an ad from an outfit in Pennsylvania that said they would pay five dollars for every hundred used tennis balls sent to them; they even provided special mailing bags. The problem with John's embrace of this wonderful idea was that he was saving the tennis balls, but he'd never gotten around to writing away for the special mailing bags. There was a closet along one wall of the tiny apartment on 67th Street where we lived together before we were married that was already full of wonderful mementos of John's Army Reserve days—including the old never-been-washed uniforms he wore to the Saturday Reserve meetings at which he ran the mimeograph machine—our winter clothes and any sports equipment either of us owned. Whatever space was left was, unbeknown to me, fast being filled by tennis balls. I wasn't aware of this plan to make us rich on used tennis balls because I had no reason to get anything out of the closet that warm spring. But I did notice pillow cases disappearing from our laundry and mentioned this to John, who said, "Oh, no, Nini, they're not lost; I'm keeping tennis balls in them."

"And where are you keeping the tennis balls?" I asked.

"Come over here; I'll show you." He opened the sliding closet door, and it was immediately obvious that whatever usefulness the pillowcases had had in keeping his collection in order had been over long ago. I'd never seen so many tennis balls. They rolled out of the closet, bouncing their way across the living-room rug, into the kitchen; their propulsion was so great that a few of them made it all the way back to our bedroom.

"Oh, John. Oh, John."

He looked at me sheepishly. I couldn't help crinkling my eyes and rolling them around a little, and he knew that was the all-clear.

"I don't believe this," I said. "Didn't you ever ask that company to send you the mailing bags?"

"I forgot, Nini," his grin huge.

"When do you think you'll write away for those bags?"

"Oh," he said slowly, "I don't know, Nini. I kind of thought I should save up a few more balls."

"What? More? There isn't room for any more."

"But Nini, they need to be sent in even hundreds to get the five dollars."

"Can't you send a few hundred out now? Jesus, John, where'd you get all these tennis balls? They can't all be yours."

"Don't worry, Nini. Here, just help me get them back into the closet."

We lived with those tennis balls for a few more months. John finally wrote away for the mailing bags, which were so small that only about twenty-five tennis balls could fit in them. That deflated his enthusiasm for this company somewhat. He had thought the bags would be the same size as pillow cases. He made a number of trips to the post office on Lexington Avenue with those small, odd, bumpy bags until he came home one night with astounding news.

"Nini, I don't think I'm going to mail the rest of these tennis balls."

"What? Why, Bunky?"

"I'll tell you, Nini," he said, his arm around my shoulder as he started walking us up and down the living room. I looked up at how much taller he was, how high his face was above me, and I listened very carefully, as he seemed about to divulge a great truth. "It's the mail clerks. They are definitely not fellow tennis-ball collectors. Nini, they're suspicious. They are not totally convinced it's tennis balls that these bags hold. I explained the great deal of the refund to one guy today. He was a great guy, too—told me about the machinery in back there, the sorters and everything—but all he said to me when he looked at the bags was, 'That's an awful lot of tennis balls.'"

By the beginning of summer the tennis-ball collection had dwindled to a more manageable size, and we had a twenty-dollar refund from the company, but as John and I made plans to move into the new apartment we had bought, and as he discussed with his friend Tom the date of the move and the time we could pick up the U-Haul, I got the definite impression the tennis balls were moving with us. I waited for an appropriate time to bring the matter up, and once I did John was surprised at my reluctance to move the balls up to 87th Street.

"But you're not using them—you're not even going to send them to Pennsylvania. Why are we hanging on to them?"

"But Nini, I saw a tennis can in Feron's that can put the pressure back into the balls. Just think, I'll never have to buy tennis balls again."

Through relatives and friends we were given that Christmas six or seven pressure cans. All different brands. Not one of them worked. I finally started throwing the tennis balls out, and by Memorial Day weekend 1975 our car had fewer than thirty tennis balls riding in the trunk with us. John was always too fast for me, though, and by the time of his death he had a new collection on the top shelf of his closet. I even saved one can of them, and my son and Leo, the cat, now play with them.

Near the end of our 1975 Bayberries summer, John and I were lying in bed, and I asked if we could start a baby. He liked the idea very much but said, "Let's wait until September, after I get my raise and have a better idea of my standing in my class at the firm." That seemed very sensible, so we waited, and the news in September was that John had gotten the highest raise in his class, and his work in the tax department was judged to be good. I had to learn early that in a law firm "good" when used to describe one's work is the equivalent of "outstanding" in regular life. So we began trying to make a baby. And right off it seemed we were lucky.

I just had a feeling I was pregnant. My worry was the hemorrhaging. Eighteen days of it. I kept calling my doctor, who thought I probably wasn't pregnant, as it was so early, and that the hemorrhaging was merely a prolonged period. And the next month I'd have a regular menstrual cycle. A couple of days later I was so weak and in such pain at a school meeting (I had a new job in my old school, Nightingale–Bamford) that I had to be walked home. I called the doctor from the bed, saying I was dizzy and in pain, and that the bleeding hadn't stopped, and I was sure I was pregnant, and he again said it didn't seem to be much to worry about, but if on Monday I felt the same, I could come in to see him, and he'd give me some hormones to stop the bleeding. I asked if I could possibly see him right then, but he said he didn't have the time.

This was a Thursday. By Saturday night, after eating brunch with John and walking home, unsteady and hurting, and having later cooked and eaten dinner, I threw up and doubled over in piercing, stabbing abdominal pain. I have never felt anything like that spear of fire. And then there was much more blood. I felt I was losing my insides. John, furious that my doctor had ignored my calls, called him and was told by the answering service that another doctor, Dr. Uscher, was on duty and that he was at the hospital, but she would get a message to him for him to call as soon as he was out of the delivery room. "It's urgent," John was saying.

Dr. Uscher called, and John started to tell him what had

happened. Dr. Uscher, impatient, wanting to get the details directly from me, demanded to speak to me. With brusque, steady assurance, he asked a few questions about the symptoms and what had happened, to which I answered yes or no. He got John back on the phone and said to him, "Get her up here immediately. Go to the emergency-room entrance, and I'll meet you there."

We were stunned. I got out of bed and hurried to get dressed. John got his Blue Cross and Blue Shield cards and we headed out into the night and rain to find a cab. It was about ten o'clock and the sky that night was starless, completely black with rain. The cab ride up the West Side Highway was agony, every pothole and bump in the pavement going right through me. John asked the driver to hurry.

The Columbia-Presbyterian Medical Center emergency room on that Saturday night was a vat of humanity, noise and even food that people had brought along with them. Many were relatives, waiting to find out what had happened to a grandparent, brother, young child. It was like the subway, and I got the impression some people hung out there for days on those rows of plastic chairs bolted to the grimy floor. John and I stood in line after line, blue arrows pointing to yellow arrows to red arrows to progress only to more questions. We repeated over and over that I was there to see Dr. Uscher. Finally a nurse said, yes, she would call Dr. Uscher: "Please sit over there until he gets down. We'll call you."

A half hour went by, forty-five minutes. At last he's here, we thought, as we peered over heads to look at any face that was attached to a person wearing a white coat. Yes, it was him. They called us. He was sorry, knew we had been there a while, deliveries one after another upstairs—just left a cesarean. He and I went into one of the examining rooms. I was so frightened. I hung on to the security of my handbag and thought of the pictures of John inside, which gave me faith and strength.

"Gee, not much blood here. Is it this side that hurts?"

"Yes."

"Does the other side hurt, too?"

"Yes."

I could see he didn't believe me, and I felt a frantic rise of fear. Then he told me he needed a urine sample. I gave one, and he walked out of the room with it saying, "I'll be back in a few minutes."

Ten minutes went by, twenty-five, a half hour. I was near crazy. Interns opened the door and went out again. "I'm waiting for Dr. Uscher," I'd say. John must have been desperate, too. When would I get out of there?

Dr. Uscher back at last: "We had to do the pregnancy test a few times, kept breaking the glass tubes. That's why I was so long." He was nice now, he was no longer ordering me to relax, damn it, as he examined me, as he had done earlier. "You're pregnant," he said.

I was wild with joy. "Really? I knew it!"

"But it's almost certain the pregnancy is in the tube." (Tube, tube, what's that? I thought desperately—I knew nothing of my own interior.) "One of your fallopian tubes," in which, as I learned later, a pregnancy cannot survive, and its growth causes the tube to burst. "How do you feel? Let's go out to John."

He told John what his suspicions were. Asked me, "Do you want to go home?" I told him it was better waiting there than here. He then looked at me. "You don't look very well. Let's get you admitted right away." But as he looked at the clock, he saw it was quarter to twelve, and he said if I were admitted now, we would have to pay for the full day. He said we still had time; we could wait until after midnight.

I went off to the ladies' room. I was so scared that for the first time in my life I learned the literal meaning of being scared shitless. Diarrhea, blood, I was pouring. I threw up. Filthy, awful, depressing ladies' room. What was happening to me fit right in. Finally I washed my face. I went back out. Dr. Uscher looked at me, and I heard I was going upstairs right away. "She could go into shock."

More questions and then forms to fill out at the admitting desk, but at least it was after midnight. John did the forms as Dr. Uscher took me up immediately. I was put in a bed in a labor room, my clothes put in a plain brown paper bag—the same kind of paper bag John's belongings were brought to me in after his death. Wedding rings and the gold necklace John had given me in St. Thomas had to be taken off. I'm losing everything, I thought to myself. I am not strong enough for this. I am a coward.

John was still downstairs filling out forms. Dr. Uscher came into the room again to get the full story *again* about my doctor's inattention to this, to the twenty days of bleeding. He was shocked. He was disgusted. Then residents, interns, each asked for details, medical history; nurses took blood samples.

John finally arrived as one of them was taking another blood sample. He flinched. This was real. This was happening to his Little One. "How do you feel, Nini? Everything'll be all right, Nini."

Dr. Uscher back fast. Did my shoulders hurt? Did it hurt when I laughed? Yes, I suddenly realized. Oh, God. What is this? Blood was moving up into the diaphragm. Now just waiting, an hour or more with John there with me until Dr. Uscher told him to go home to get some rest, that he promised he would call before he operated. Then an intern in to put in the IV. Now I was alone. I say I'm Rh-negative. He ran out of the room, and said over his shoulder, "Good you said that." Back in. He first tried to get the needle into the back of my left hand. It wouldn't go in. He jabbed. My hand started turning black and blue. He was nervous; I told him to take his time. Somehow I was now incredibly calm, and I just wanted him to relax and do it right. Finally the IV was in the back of my right hand.

Another hour alone. Nothing to do, nothing to read, no radio for music. Depressing green room, window so filthy that I couldn't see out of it. Hard lights and a school clock with a second hand. I heard women panting and breathing in labor rooms down the hall. Even then I had started to become jealous of the alive babies they would take home. "Okay," I heard out in the hall, "Mrs. B——, you're going into the delivery room now; you're ten centimeters dilated. You're doing just fine." And the husband, "Here we go. You're doing fine, Sue, just fine. I'm right here. We've got forty-five seconds until the next one." Contraction, that is. What I was hearing out in the hall was a team of a man and wife. Doctors pleased, all tense, expectant but happy. This will be a fast, healthy birth, they were thinking to themselves.

Dr. Uscher back. "I think we might as well let you go down to your room. You can get some sleep there." I was wheeled down on a stretcher. I was no longer a walking person—I was a lying-down patient with an IV in me, although I was still thinking of it as an intravenous tube. It wouldn't be until John's cancer that the abbreviation IV would come so quickly to my lips.

Down in my room Dr. Uscher again asked if it hurt when I laughed. My shoulders were now in great pain. He examined me and inserted a long, long, long needle up through me into my abdomen to withdraw some fluid. This was agony, incredible pain. The fluid was blood: I was hemorrhaging internally. He told the nurse whose hand I'd been holding and practically crushed under my grip of fear, "Prep her. We're going back up." Prep her? What was this? The quiet, soft, gentle Irish nurse told me,

as she whipped together lather, I was being shaved for
surgery. Oh, God. Dr. Uscher called John to let him know
that he was going to operate right away. Now shaved, I
was rolled back up to the operating room. "I'm Rh-negative," I kept repeating. Waited and waited in the operating
room.

"What's taking so long getting the blood up here? Call
them again," Dr. Uscher barked. Gloves on, masks on all.
Lots of nurses. The anesthesiologist, a woman, in a sing-
song hard-to-understand English. "Have you ever had
anesthesia before?" "Only ether when I was little for an
eye operation." I was fading. Things were losing their
sharp outline. "When did you last eat?" Food? Oh, yes,
dinner. "Eight o'clock, but I threw up at home afterward
and then again here." "Good," she said. "Let's drape her
now anyway," said Dr. Uscher. My hair was pulled back
into a paper cap, and I kept thinking how dirty it was, I
had planned to wash it in the morning.

Legs up and spread apart. Green towels went up across
my chest to prevent me from seeing. My legs shook.
"She's cold," someone said. "Put the socks on her."
White socks, funny things, big but felt like flannel. Warm.
Everything green, green tiles and stainless steel every-
where. Trays of stainless-steel instruments. I was fascinated; what is that one used for? I wondered. They were
all impatient, they wanted to get started. Finally, "Give
her the . . ."—some kind of tranquilizer. I'm going to die, I
thought. "It will make your throat dry; don't worry." One
arm strapped to the table; the other strapped to an ex-
tended board toward the Indian anesthesiologist. I still
couldn't understand her English, words ran into each
other, so musical, but impossible to understand. I felt I
was going to cry because I couldn't understand what she
was saying. "Okay, it's in, it's starting."

Relaxing peace; I was happy, calm. Mouth dry, but I

kept some spit in it because they had warned me of the dryness. I moved my tongue around in it to keep it wet. Dr. Uscher asked, "Do you ever wear bikinis?" What kind of question was that? But I said yes, when I'm thin enough. "Really?" He was skeptical. Is this kid ever thin enough? I could hear him thinking. "Okay," he said, "I'll do a bikini incision; you won't see it when you wear a bikini bathing suit." All of a sudden I was thanking all of them so earnestly. "You're all so nice," I said. I was drunk. "The blood's here." "At last." "Let's go," said Dr. Uscher. It was four-thirty in the morning.

Anesthesiologist, in her hard-to-understand English: "You're going to go to sleep now." This I had always been petrified of, so much so that when my wisdom teeth were removed, the sodium pentathol didn't work, and I had to be given nine shots of Novocain instead. But now it no longer mattered. I was in so much pain, I wanted release. I was going to die, I thought. Then the mask over my nose and mouth. "Breathe deeply." And without a blink, I was under. Blackness, gone.

Something was happening. It turned out that they were stitching me up, and I was coming out too fast, but the muscle relaxant was still working. I couldn't open my mouth, speak, or open my eyes. I wanted to scream. I thought of Joan Sutherland's wide-open mouth singing on the stage of the Met in *The Daughter of the Regiment*. I was under again. Frightening. I'll never forget it.

Seven-thirty in the morning. Awake to a blue-and-silver recovery room with Dr. Uscher right beside me. It was the most beautiful room I've ever been in, although a later operation and a baby let me see more clearly that it was just a drab, colorless room. The white sheets and the screens between the beds looked like clouds. I was in a silver and blue and white cloud room. I was alive.

"It was a tubal pregnancy. You'd lost a lot of blood, but

we didn't have to give you a transfusion. I had to take the tube—the fetus had burst it—but I left the ovary. It's the left-side tube—*your* left side," he said as he looked down at me. My mouth moved and said thank you. He didn't understand my gratefulness was for being alive. He'd saved my life, it seemed. I learned later that tubal pregnancies are life-threatening.

I was back downstairs in my room. "Oh, Nini, you're all right," said John. "Oh, I love you so much, Nini. I went home to change clothes. When I left here, I took your raincoat with me and got on the subway. I took it down to Columbus Circle and walked home through the park, carrying your raincoat." This at three in the morning. I was frightened for the danger he'd put himself in, to walk through the park at that hour on a November night. "And when I got home, Nini, I went into the bedroom, and the closet door was open, and there was your blue shirt, your workshirt, and I took it out and held it to my face and cried and cried. I was so afraid something was going to happen to the Little One. I was so afraid I was going to lose you. Then Dr. Uscher called and said they were going to operate. He's a wonderful man, Nini. Oh, Nini, I love you so much, Nini."

After the joy of being alive, a few days later I fell into the deepest depression. The incision hurt so—so much it can't be described. I walked bending over—nurses forced me to stand up straight. And I heard the depression was partly due to the abrupt end of a pregnancy and of all the hormone production of the beginning weeks. The fetus had been seven weeks old. Already I missed it and wanted it back.

One morning a nurse came in at six with a baby, a dear curled-up pink newborn. She was surprised I was not ready.

"Good morning. It's time to feed your baby."

Groggily, "I, ah, don't have a baby." She looked at me thinking this one had gone off the deep end.

"Yes, *here's* your baby."

"No, this is a mistake. I'm here because I had an ectopic pregnancy. I don't *have* a baby!" Her arms loosened their hold on the pink newborn and almost let him go.

"Oh, my God," she said, and rushed out of the room. "I'm sorry," she stammered over her shoulder.

Then John and I leaving the day I was discharged. Went down in the elevator in a wheelchair, handled by a young man. A few of his friends got on the elevator at a lower floor and said hi to him, and knowing he was coming down with me from the maternity floor, they asked me, "Where's your baby?" I was holding a plant in my lap.

"I didn't have a baby. Maybe next time." Shots of hurt pierced through me.

One day as John was visiting me in my room at the hospital, I jokingly asked him, couldn't I *now* have a cat? He didn't like them at all and had adamantly refused in the past.

"Yes, Nini, of course, Nini." Then weeks later when I reminded him of it he said, "Do you really want a cat? Let's not get one."

"Okay, Bunky." It became a party joke for a long time. "Here I chose the perfect time to ask John for a cat, and he said yes, and then once I got home, he said no!" Only after a year of infertility did we get our cat, which John adored, although he could barely admit it; I'd catch him once in a while holding and cuddling Leo, murmuring soft words to him.

The weekend he finally agreed that I could get a cat we went from pet store to pet store in the car looking for a Burmese kitten. Finally went to a place on the West Side called the Cat Cottage. It turned out they sold only cat equipment: leashes, collars, coats, hats, rubbers, sleeping nests, pagoda beds! However, when we asked if they knew where we could get a Burmese, the answer was yes. The owner knew a woman in Brooklyn who bred Burmese cats, and there had been a recent litter. Her name was Joan Fogarty, and they gave us her telephone number.

When we got home, John said, "Here's her number; why don't you call her up?" I said, "No, you call her."

As he dialed the number, I started to giggle, and then when Joan answered, I heard John say, "Hi, Joan, my name's John Rossi, I got your name at a cat house on the West Side." John didn't realize what he'd said. I was on the floor. I was laughing, soundlessly, so hard I couldn't even straighten out. "Yes, my wife and I are looking for a Burmese cat, and we were told by the people at the cat house that you had some for sale. . . . Okay, we'll be out tomorrow. Let me write down the directions. . . . Here, I've got a pencil now"—which I'd staggered off to find for him; John thought I'd truly gone bonkers. "Yes, yes. . . . Okay, I think I've got it. We'll be out after one o'clock tomorrow then. Goodbye."

"Oh, John, do you know what you said? You said you got her name at a *cat house* on the West Side!"

"Oh, my God, Nini. I thought she sounded a little strange at first. Did I really say that?"

"Yes—you meant the Cat *Cottage*." He fell to the floor on top of me laughing as hard as I had.

John then would go on to tell the story to others of how we went out to Flatbush to Joan's apartment, which, he said, was at least 90 degrees inside, and he described the place. "Cats on the opened couch bed in the living room. That's their bed, explains Joan. Cats all over the place. There are bookshelves all across one wall of the living room with the books on their sides, and the bindings facing the wall, pages to the room! How does she know how to find a book?" Disbelief and wide-eyed fascination would cross his face as he continued and started to describe Joan's boyfriend. "Her boyfriend, Henry, is there. He also breeds cats, and he's there to pick out a female. His back is permanently bent over, with his arms dangling at his sides, reaching his shoes, from leaning over to pick up so many goddam cats. I couldn't wait to get out of there, but Nini had to spend over an hour there deciding on the right cat!"

As I held each little kitten—six of them, some of them dark brown and some champagne-colored—John in his inimitable way found out all he could about Joan's and Henry's lives, why they bred cats, where they worked.

I saw a little kitten asleep on my coat and figured what the hell, he must want to come home with me. Joan said I'd picked the best one; he had spunk. She didn't tell us he was also incredibly dumb, which he is. He is the only cat I've known who trips over his own feet. We got a cardboard box, paid Joan 150 dollars by check, while John practically fainted, and Joan said, "Wait, let me look for the pedigree papers; he's of a champion line."

"Don't worry, Joan," said John, "send them to us." He wanted out fast.

As we drove over the Manhattan Bridge, I asked John what we should name him. "Leo," he said with complete sincerity. So Leo it was.

We had always seen Dr. Uscher at his office at Columbia-Presbyterian, but because this month was so crucial, he had us come out this afternoon to his office in Tenafly, New Jersey. The appointment didn't take very long. The good news was that John's sperm count was more than average and that the sperm looked perfectly normal. Dr. Uscher wasn't surprised. So he announced that this month during the days around ovulation he was going to give me a pill called Premarin to improve the currently inhospitable acidic mucus in my cervix. So for the next weeks we were on a schedule to make love every other day, and keep track of it on the temperature chart (which he'd had us do for months anyway). I remember one morning—sometimes we'd make love in the morning before we went to his Columbia office for our seven-thirty appointment—when he looked at our chart and saw that we'd made love that morning and also that we'd made love more than we "had" to, he smiled and winked. He said, "I've been looking at your temperature charts for months now, and I've got to tell you, you two have the best sex life of any of my patients." John and I grinned.

And it worked. I was pregnant and knew it early because my temperature on the chart remained over 98 degrees for days, and my period hadn't started, and besides, I just knew. I was so excited and couldn't wait until enough time had passed so that I could have a real pregnancy test.

I called up Dr. Uscher, and he said, "I knew it. I knew when I didn't hear from you two that we must have hit the jackpot. Now let's see, let me get out your chart here. I gave you the Premarin on the seventeenth, eighteenth and nineteenth of April, right? And, yeah, I'm just looking at this, sure, you ovulated on the nineteenth for sure. And your temperature's still high, right? Give me the numbers for each day up to now so I can fill them in. Okay. Well, it's still awfully early for the urine test, but you've got that lab down near you. Why don't you drop off a specimen there anyway, yeah, drop it off tomorrow morning. Remember, it's a sample of the first urine when you wake up."

I wrote that down and then kept thanking him over the phone and told him how happy John and I were. And he said, "Well, let's wait till the test tomorrow, but it sure looks pretty certain. And don't be too upset if it's negative;

we'll just wait another week and do it again. Don't worry; I'll call you as soon as the lab calls me tomorrow."

Which he did. It was negative, and I thought I was going to fold up with disappointment and despair. I couldn't help it. But he said he was still sure I was pregnant and that the next week we would repeat the test but have it done at the lab at the hospital. He was not too crazy about the lab near me anyway. I dreaded John's coming home from work that evening, because I knew I would cry and he would ask why, and I would tell him about the negative test result. On top of everything he had to leave for a business trip to Europe the day after, so he wouldn't even be there when I had the second test. I didn't want to go through it alone.

I know this all must seem pretty minor and silly, but infertility and the desperate desire for a baby are such unhappy, lonely times for a couple to go through. It becomes a subject always floating around the two of you but is discussed less and less after all the tests have been done, all the medical advice taken. You even start to believe that maybe, yes, it's in your head. Maybe you really don't want a baby, and you *know* that's not true, but you start to consider it, because maybe something a doctor or nurse said to you implied that he or she thought that, and the whole thing makes you crazy. It takes a special marriage and a special doctor to understand the thin tightwire of hope and despair that is a part of every month of the year, year after year. What with the temperature charts, you know when you ovulate, so you're hoping for the two weeks after that that maybe this month, maybe you won't get your period, maybe you'll finally be pregnant.

What's really cruel is when the days go by, and maybe just because of the strain of your hoping your period is a few days late, so you start being extra-careful with yourself: no running or jogging, no climbing stairs even, because this might be it, and you don't want anything to go wrong. In the last days before your period eventually does arrive, you even decide to cut out any coffee or liquor just in case you are pregnant. It is absurd, and you don't even tell your husband why you're not going out jogging with him. You make up an excuse. But he's not dumb, and a week later when he sees you come out of the bathroom, looking as though you've been crying, with your face all pulled back and a couple of tampons in your hand to put in your purse for when you're at the office, he knows.

John would say, "You got your period, huh, Little One?" And I'd say, "Yeah," real quietly. He'd sit me down on the bed before leaving for work and say, "You *know* this means as much to me as it does to you, but Little One, you've got to remember you're the one I love. It isn't that I don't care if we never have a baby, I do care, but it's just that you are so much more important to me. All I want is for you to be happy. I love you so much. Please don't let it get you down too much today. I want to see the happy, frisky Nini when I come home tonight. You just don't know what you mean to me, Little One, and when you're sad, I'm sad. Come on, give me a kiss. Now, chin up. Let's see a smile—remember, 'great in '78,' that's what the Little One's going to be. Please don't worry, Nancy, everything's going to be okay. And just think," and he'd say this shyly, not with bravado, but shyly, "just think, Nini, you've got me."

"Oh, Bunky. I know. I love you so much. I'll cheer up. I promise. It throws me. I don't know why. I think I've forgotten about it, that I am living my life happily just as it is, and then another period comes, and I lose all perspective. I'm sorry, Bunky. You're the only person I can talk to, and I know it's hard on you, too. I don't know what I'd do without you. You always can cheer me up." And he would start making funny faces. "Yep," he'd say, as he started to see me smile, "there's my Nini. You have a good day at school today, beautiful, okay? I hope you're working on the Island of Borneo play with the fifth grade."

"Oh, no, John. That was a couple of years ago; you know that."

"Sure, I know, but I wish you'd do it again, 'cause I missed it the first time when I had to go to Detroit." And he'd recite, "I am the Island of Borneo, where the farmer, poor farmer, bends low, bends low." I hadn't even written it; it was out of a book, a play about the ecosystem, and it tied in with their science course. But John loved that line about the farmer bending low, and as he'd say it, he'd bend over looking sad in the face, and I'd start to laugh. "Boy," John would say, "that's just the way I feel in the subway. There's nothing like being packed on the Lexington Avenue express on a sunny morning to make you feel like you're bending low, bending low. Just thinking about it depresses me. I'm going to walk to work. I'd better get going. Now listen, Nini, you be a good girl today and don't run off with Robert Redford, because I want to chase you around the apartment when I get home, and I'm worried if Redford's here, you might rather run after him. So please, Nini, no matter how many times he calls, how much he pesters you, do not run away with him. Capisce?"

John could make up stories like that all the time. He might even call me at the office that day to make sure Redford hadn't come over for lunch in the Nightingale cafeteria. "No," I'd say, "he hasn't arrived yet." Other times he would just call in the middle of the afternoon to ask if I loved him. "Do you love me, Nini?" "Of course, Bunky, of course I do." "Good," he'd say, "I'll see you tonight." And he'd hang up. He didn't think anything of talking like that in front of others.

I never really knew why he kept asking me if I loved

him or telling me never to leave him. I never knew what he meant. Sometimes I'd ask him if he really thought I might ever leave him, is that why he talked about it? And then I'd say that of course he knew how much I loved him and that that was never going to happen. John answered once, "I don't know why I do that; I just don't ever want to lose you, that's all."

"You're never going to lose me, John; I'm always going to be with you. If anything, you're the one who's going to leave me for some nice tall skinny girl. So please don't talk about my leaving you. I know you're joking most of the time, but when you ask me so seriously, it makes me nervous."

Something else he'd do: all of a sudden while he was shaving, driving the car, running, whatever, he'd go, "Oh, no," and kind of slap his forehead, and I'd say, "Bunky, what's wrong?" And he'd say, "I just remembered something I did when I was younger. Boy, I said and did some dumb things." And I'd ask what he'd remembered that was so dumb or so awful, and he'd say, "Oh, nothing, Nini, nothing important." I'd answer, "It couldn't be that bad; you can tell me."

And sometimes he would and sometimes he wouldn't, but the times he did, the events he described seemed so insignificant to me, significant at the time certainly but not things to fret over now. Something like "Once I raised my hand in chemistry class in high school to show I knew the answer to the question the teacher'd asked, and he called on me, and, of course, I didn't know the answer; I'd just raised my hand to make it look as if I did, to look smart. So when he called on me, I had to admit I didn't know, but first I invented an answer that of course was wrong."

And I'd tell him, "Bunky, everyone's done that. Raised his hand and then surprise, surprise, the teacher actually calls on you. It's nothing to worry about now. What made you think of it, anyway? Something at the office?" And he'd screw up his face and say no, that it had just occurred to him, that's all, and then he'd repeat, "Sometimes I'm so dumb." Then I'd put my arm around him and say, "Bunky, you're not dumb. You're the smartest, most wonderful man I've ever known, and I still have to pinch myself to realize I'm really married to you. You're fantastic. Besides, I always thought you did well in chemistry. A's and B's, right?" And John would nod his head. "Probably was the only question you ever got wrong, huh? Is that the problem?"

"No," he said, "I just didn't like to look dumb. You know, Nini, I was never elected to anything in school, not like you, you know that? I was not very popular."

I was stunned. The man who was saying this was one of the best-liked people in his huge law firm; all of his friends envied his happy, easy manner. John not popular? It was a staggering piece of information.

"Oh, my social life was okay, I mean with girls. I never had any trouble there, in fact, I think some of the guys were jealous, but I just never was popular. Tom, Steve and Jim were my only friends in high school; I'd have to say that in college and law school only Mike and Phil were. I don't know, Nini, I just don't know." And he'd shake his head back and forth.

"Bunky, look, look at me, look at all the people who love you now: all the people at work, all your friends, all my friends, your family, my family, even all the cab drivers you talk to. Everyone who meets you likes you."

"I know," he'd say. "Living here in New York is the first time I've ever been popular."

I shake my head now, looking down at my seed catalogues—he should know, he should know how popular he was. He should know that his law firm set up a trust fund for our son's education to which they as a firm and all of his friends contributed, and that the firm just this spring named the tennis trophy that is won every year at their spring outing the John F. Rossi Memorial Tennis Trophy. It was about a year and a half after John's death, and I'd gotten my driver's license at last the previous summer at age thirty. The law firm had sent me invitations to their annual winter dinner and spring outing after John died, but I had felt I could not go, feared it would be too difficult for me, too full of memories. But this past June they asked particularly that I come up and at least spend the day at the country club, said that I could bring the baby, and that we could swim and that everyone would be so happy to see him and me. After deciding that, yes, I could do that, and that it would probably be fun, I accepted. Then I was urged to stay for the dinner and dance that followed. It would be no trouble, they said. Sheryl said she had a baby-sitter already lined up for her own children and that John could stay there and then we could both spend the night so that I wouldn't have to drive back into the city late at night. As with many things I've done since John's death, I said yes at every turn until I suddenly realized that I was in fact going to the outing and staying for the dinner and the dance.

It was a nice warm day. In the car on the way up I played some good music on the tape deck, some Carly Simon particularly, as she always makes me think of summers with John, and for today at least I had to think of him and get some strength from that, and with the map on my lap I managed to find the place. It sure hadn't changed much, the Apawamis Club. I can remember how I was shaking when I parked the car in the parking lot, and an older gentleman asked me if this was the right place, if this was where the Kelley Drye outing was, and I, as if I were still John's wife, still the one who'd done the decorating of the dining room as I'd done in the past a couple of times, still the wife of the man who always did the seating assignments, still a member of the Kelley Drye community, authoritatively answered, "Oh, yes, this is the place." Then he asked me for directions to the clubhouse and the tennis courts, and I said, "Well, if I remember correctly, just go up that hill, follow the driveway around the corner, and you'll be in front of the clubhouse. The tennis courts are off to the side in back."

This is unreal, I thought, as I unstrapped my son from his car seat. The man then introduced himself and his wife. I'd never heard their names before; he was new at Kelley Drye, in the accounting department, so he didn't recognize my name either when I told him. "See you later," I said and waved to them. Unbelievable. Jesus, John, I thought, why the hell aren't you here with me?

After getting out all our stuff and locking the car, I put John into the stroller and walked up to the clubhouse and out to the back, off to the side, to the tennis courts and the pool. Everyone was grouped at tables in tennis clothes watching the tennis game closest to the patio. Immediately I was recognized, and there was much fussing and oohing and aahing over the baby. And, "How well you look, Nancy, you look just great. So this is John. He's beautiful. More beautiful than his pictures. What a handsome boy. Looks just like you. Oh, look, he's walking and everything. Here, come over here, John, and sit by me. What would you like, Nancy? Have you two eaten lunch? Let me get you something."

I answered, "No, that's all right. I'll just go over to the snack bar and get John and me a sandwich. Would you look after him for me?"

"Oh, sure," they said.

I had to get away for a few moments. I walked up to the outdoor hamburger-sandwich bar, and didn't even know what I was ordering. How incredibly nice everyone was being to me and John. As I learned quickly after John's death, it is people's kindness and caring that make me want to cry, that in a funny way make me feel loneliest. I felt overwhelmed but also, quickly, amazingly comfortable. It was like being back home even though John wasn't there, and the rest of the afternoon passed delightfully, seeing and talking to old friends, and when it was time for the dinner that evening, I was very glad I'd come after all. As dinner was ending, though, I knew the hardest part of the day was about to come. It was going to be another "first" to get through.

You see, John had always run the tennis tournament, and he was the one who had announced the winners and handed out the trophy and the prizes after dinner. I wondered how I was going to be able to sit at my table and watch anyone else do it. I was even all ready to get up to go to the ladies' room and sort of hide in there, but before I could get away, the two friends of John's who were going to handle the tennis and golf awards came up to me and very quietly told me that it had been decided to name the tennis trophy for John and would it be all right if they announced it that night? They said they understood if I'd prefer they didn't announce it while I was there, that it might be too emotional for me and that they could announce it at the firm at a later date, but what did I think? They'd do whatever made me most comfortable.

At first my reaction was no, they can't announce it tonight, I can't stand it, it would be too much and surely I'd cry because it showed such kindness. But in talking it over with them, I quickly reconsidered. No, this honor should be announced tonight. I said, though, that instead of sitting conspicuously at the table I was at, I'd rather watch it and hear it from backstage so to speak. So I went out to the hallway alongside the dining room with another friend of

John's, someone to give me courage, and I told him what they were going to do and asked if he would just stand there with me in the hallway. He understood and said sure.

I could see things starting to bustle inside, the men nodding their heads. "Yes," I overheard, "she's agreed." They all looked very pleased. The two men went up to the microphones set up for announcing the winners, and even as I struggled to keep my feet firmly and bravely on the floor underneath me, I was also incredibly proud. My John. They were doing this for my John. This was something our son would know about one day. What fine, fine people. Everyone clapped. It was over, and it hadn't been somber at all. I'd had nothing to worry about. Everyone was very happy, was smiling.

A senior partner came over to me and put it beautifully. He said, "We wanted to do something for John, more than just money; we wanted him to be remembered. We thought that years from now when a young associate wins this trophy and asks, 'Who on earth was John Rossi?' he would hear the story."

And Bunky saying he wasn't popular as a kid. Whew.

Well, John did go off to Europe on his business trip before the second pregnancy test. He had to go to London, Coventry, Paris and Madrid. It was the second time he'd gone to Europe for the firm, but this was the first time he'd gone alone. He was very proud. There aren't that many things that I have of John's, but he did write me one poem and this letter.

MAY 9, 1978
6 P.M.
HOTEL MERIDIEN, PARIS

Dear Nini,
Do you love me? I love you. I have now had some time to

walk around Paris but will not be able to see any museums. The weather has been overcast, but the temperature has been around 50°—just perfect for me.

So far, the trip has not been a head-high stack of hits, but I am eating very well. Yesterday I had salad Nicoise (sp?) for lunch.

I hope you are still great in '78, and I miss you very much. I would particularly like to see you with your lower lip sticking out.

Like a good boy I have written postcards to Diane, Suzanne, my mother, Linuccia, and Granny.

The plan is still to go to London tomorrow afternoon and to Madrid on the 17th.

I really wish you could have come with me, but we will take a nice long trip together soon (when we save the money).

I would be overjoyed if you are really pregnant, but I am overjoyed with you anyway so, in a sense, it doesn't make any difference to me. So do not get depressed because I intend to put you on the platform when I get back.

> *I love you very much.*
> *Love,*
> *John*

On May 16 I went to the hospital alone for the test. I went first thing in the morning, before school, and as I walked out the door, I gave Leo, the cat, a hug and scratched him under his chin and said to him, "Keep your fingers crossed, Leo." I got to the lab by eight o'clock and left the urine specimen. Dr. Uscher again said he would call me as soon as he had the results, and I'd promised to call John by six that evening. I got back to school and before lunch Uscher called. I was most certainly pregnant. My God.

I was so happy and grateful I floated the rest of the day. I remember I was taking minutes at a school meeting, and before it began I'd told my friend who was running it that I'd have to leave by five-thirty so that I could make my call to John in Madrid, and I whispered to her, "I'm pregnant." She beamed; she was six months pregnant herself. "I found out today, and John's in Europe, and I promised I'd call." So at five-thirty, I excused myself and walked the five blocks home as if I were the most special creature on earth. Certainly the happiest. I got off the elevator and was so excited I could barely hold the keys. I couldn't wait to get to that telephone. I got the door open, and ran past Leo there in the front hall, greeting me as always, and said to him, "We did it, Leo, we did it!"

I carefully placed the call, and the seconds went by so slowly, first talking to the international operator and then listening to her talk to the Spanish operator and then the hotel operator and then finally hearing them ring John's room. It rang once, twice, and then I heard John pick it up and say hello.

"John, John," I said.

"Nini, oh, Nini, it's so good to hear your voice."

"John, we did it! I'm pregnant! I'm really pregnant. The test was fine. I see Uscher first thing tomorrow morning."

"Oh, Little One, oh, Nini," and his voice choked a little, "I'm so happy. I love you so much. When's it due?"

"January eleventh, next January, 1979."

"I wish I were right there with you. But listen, you take care, you take care of yourself, Little One, and I'll see you Saturday. Sleep tight. I love you." And we hung up.

John came home, and I don't think I've ever been so happy to see anyone in my life. We talked about the pregnancy, and I wanted to hear about his trip, and he said it wasn't much to shout about, that he'd been pretty busy working, but he said, "Oh, wait a minute, I forgot. Last

week when I was in the Palace Hotel in Madrid, I wanted
to have breakfast delivered to my room, so I looked over
the menu and saw they had hot cereal. You know I like
porridge. Well, when the waiter rolled in my breakfast, I
saw a bowl of cornflakes. I pointed to them and said, 'No,
hot, hot cereal, not cold.' The waiter shook his head and
didn't understand, so I took him into the bathroom and
turned on the hot water in the sink and said, 'Hot, Hot.'
And then I put my hand under the hot water, and said,
'Hot,' and the waiter still didn't understand, so I put his
hand under the water and again said, 'Hot, hot cereal.' He
then took me by the hand back to the breakfast tray and
poured a pitcher of milk over the cornflakes and then put
my hand in the bowl and said, 'Hot.' The milk that was in
the pitcher was hot milk! So that's hot cereal in Madrid.
See, Nini, you learn something every day."

A few days went by, and I didn't feel so hot. For one
thing I had started to bleed, and it threw me right back to
that first ectopic pregnancy. Dr. Uscher said there was a 95
percent chance the pregnancy was developing normally in
the uterus and not in the tube. The least bit of uncertainty,
though, made me feel blue and unsure of myself. This
pregnancy just had to be successful. I didn't know how I
would deal with another ectopic, and I got so afraid that I
started to believe that I had better not hope for the good,
because if it all came crashing down, if it was another
ectopic, I would have farther to fall and farther to struggle
up again. Could I really hope? I knew I was too anxious. I
reminded myself that I must remember others I had heard
about whose first pregnancy was a tubal one and who
then went on to have children. I wondered how Julie
Eisenhower got through these first weeks. Was she as
worried and as scared as I was? The memory of the sudden surprise of the last time and the horrible pain kept me
in suspense. Could I dare go out to Bridgehampton that

weekend? If I could just get through another couple of weeks, I thought, I would know I didn't have this to fear. And I recalled a sentence from one of Anne Morrow Lindbergh's books: "I do not know why we all live counting on the laws of Chance, when it is always the exception that affects our lives." I was thinking how perfectly that fit me right then when I was praying I wouldn't lose that baby.

So when I next talked to Dr. Uscher and he asked about the bleeding, he said, enough is enough, and that I should come to the hospital for a sonogram before Memorial Day weekend so that we could find out for sure if the bleeding could possibly be caused by an imminent ectopic. Thank God, at least this time John was there to go with me. It seemed that for months we had set the alarm early, rolled out of bed and raced up to that hospital by the George Washington Bridge. We could tell you exactly how far along they were—not very—on their work to improve the West Side Highway. And we were there so often that the security guard at Atchley Pavilion waved to us.

We went to Dr. Uscher's office, and he told us where to go in the hospital, where the sonogram lab was. We went winding back through Harkness and Presbyterian and up in the elevator to the eighteenth floor. What was so striking about Presbyterian was how old and grungy it was and yet there were nice wooden doors to all the rooms. The hallway outside the sonogram room was depressing, and it didn't look as if it had even been cleaned and mopped in a long time. But when the technician opened the door and asked me to come in, we entered a room with the most modern space-age equipment. Such a contrast: funny old plaster walls and ceiling fixtures and the old wooden doors and linoleum floors and in the middle of it was an X-ray machine with a television screen.

The technician asked to make sure I'd drunk at least

eight glasses of water before coming over. Yes, I answered, I had. A full bladder would push the uterus into a
better viewing position for the sonogram. She kept asking
me if I was sure I had had enough water, and I assured her
I had. While John waited outside I got undressed and into
a hospital gown and then lifted myself up onto the examining table. She then lifted the gown and poured some
sticky substance over my stomach. She warned me that it
would feel icy, and it did. Then she attached a couple of
small discs with wires attached to them, and then she
poured more lotion on and turned on the video screen. In
her right hand she had what looked like a strange-shaped
microphone, and she began moving it slowly over my
stomach, looking at the screen as she did it. I wasn't
scared at all. I was fascinated, and she told me to turn my
head back so that I could look at the screen, too.

"We'll see the baby's head soon. Oh, there it is, see?
Oh, everything's fine. Yes, it's in the uterus. And what,
you're about seven weeks? Looks normal to me. There,
now look, I'll keep it here for a moment, see the baby's
heart, it's still pretty much outside the chest cavity, but
you can sure see it beating, can't you? And you see the
arms and legs? Still really like flippers, although you can
see the beginning of the digits. And look at the eyes." She
had been pointing her finger to different places on the
screen.

This was my baby. I breathed quietly. I was in awe.
Here on a television screen I was seeing the miracle of life,
the existence of God. Forget my wedding, forget my con-
firmation at the Cathedral of St. John the Divine, forget
even Christmas Eve pageants and services, this was religion. To watch this television screen and see another
generation, a generation unborn.

I repeated, "It's not in the tube."

"No," the technician reassured me, "it's in the uterus.

Perfectly normal." I was crying, and she said, "This really means a lot to you, doesn't it?"

"Oh, yes," I said, "my husband and I have tried for so long."

She said, "Here, I'll go out and tell your husband the news." The screen was black now. She had turned it off, taken the sterile gloves off her hands, and I was left alone looking at a cracking ceiling. I heard her call out that I could get dressed and I could also go to the bathroom and pee now, thank goodness. I could hear John's voice. He sounded so happy.

It was so still, though. A quiet hospital room with such private joy within its walls. I thanked God for the miracle. I was going to have a baby, and I had seen it! I had seen the ears, the nose, the face, the little, tiny, curled body all floating in me. Once when the technician passed the soundwave microphone near its foot it jerked it even. The baby. So lucky I was. I couldn't wait to get out to John, but strangely I was comforted and tranquil and wanted these few moments alone to let what I had just seen sink in quietly.

John came in, followed by the technician. I zipped up my skirt and peeked around the corner of the curtained dressing room and looked at him. What a smile he had on his face. I came out and hugged him, buried my face in his neck high above me. The technician was really in the spirit of things, and she said, "Come on into my office. Let's call Dr. Uscher and tell him."

So we went in and she dialed his number, and he answered, and she said, "Hi, Dr. Uscher, I think I have the happiest two people in the world here. Yes, the Rossis, how did you guess? Well, everything's fine, the fetus is developing normally in the uterus. I'll send over the pictures when they're developed. Yes, I'll tell them, yeah, they really are happy."

We took the elevator back down, walked back through the hospital and went back to our car. It had been about an hour and a half that we had been there, and we were both going to be late for work. John kept hugging me and I kept hugging him. John said, "I just knew it was good news, I heard you and the technician in there practically crying, but happy crying."

"That was me, that's for sure," I said. "I just wish you could have come in to see it on the screen. You can't imagine what it was like. I really saw *our* baby!"

"Could you tell if it was a boy or a girl?" he asked.

"No, I couldn't. I don't know. I wonder if the technician could, and she just didn't say anything. It's probably too early to tell, though. I really wouldn't want to know, though, would you?" And John agreed that no, he wouldn't want to know either. "A lot more exciting, I think, to wait and find out when it's born," I said.

We got into the car and took our usual route back downtown on Riverside Drive, a lot less traffic than on the by now rush-hour West Side Highway. We were talking all the way, and we didn't even realize we had missed the turn-off for 96th Street to get us back to the garage near our house. John was so excited that everything was okay. We were so happy, we laughed at our mistake.

Oh boy, we thought, this is the top: finally a baby, a family, our marriage, his success at Kelley Drye and being up for partnership this year, my work at school, our home in New York City, our house in Long Island. It had been so much work, and now we had been granted our greatest wish, to be parents. We called all our family that night and told them.

CHAPTER THREE

The day had started at seven, John off to play tennis with his friend Tony Schlesinger and me to check the overnight growth of weeds in the vegetable garden and make an attempt to pull out as many of the invading forces as possible before the sun got too hot on my back, and then in to make sandwiches to take down to the beach, the iced tea—a beer for John—and to be ready when he got back at nine-thirty. It was July 1978. Over my bathing suit I wore a Mexican shirt I'd had since college, and I smiled, remembering that a boy I knew at the University of Colorado used to call this shirt my "hatching jacket," said that certainly under the many pleated folds falling from the yoke around the neck I must be hatching something, and I looked down at a stomach that was just starting to protrude and thanked God that at last I was hatching something.

I heard the car pull into the driveway, and John, dripping, mopping his face with a towel, came in, saying,
"Give me a kiss, Nini." His brown curly hair bushed out
from under the blue terry tennis headband in the humidity, his tennis shirt stuck to his body, the shirttail hanging
out over his shorts as always, and after patting me on my
head, he went upstairs to get into his favorite bathing suit,
a pair of faded, well-washed cotton trunks in a tattersall
print of gray, black and pink lines on a white background;
we had bought them on sale a couple of years ago, and he
liked those pink lines. I shouted up the staircase to ask
him how about putting the dirty tennis clothes into the
hamper instead of leaving them in a pile on the floor, you
know, just for a change, waddya think? "Oh, Nini," I hear
from above, "now what fun would that be? Our room
needs a little floor decoration." We laughed. I wasn't surprised; we had been playing this game for too many years
now: I left my shoes on the floor where we always tripped
over them, and he dumped tennis and running clothes in
a heap. This from a man who actually loved to vacuum
and do the laundry, as long as he didn't have to fold it.

He came down the stairs, carrying a book, and picked
up the cooler, and we headed out to the car. "You've got
my sunglasses, Little One?"

"Yep."

We drove down Ocean Road. Looked like the roadside
stand had started to get some corn in; we would have to
buy some on our way back. The wind blew through the
windows of Mom's orange 1970 Volkswagen. There was a
new house going up on Dune Road, ugly; last week there
were just posts in the ground, this week the wooden skel-
eton gave us some idea of the final design—awful. We felt
we owned this stretch of Dune Road, ever since we had
seen Woody Allen and Diane Keaton driving down it in
Annie Hall, and, our minds thinking of the same thing,

John said, "Remember that part in *Love and Death* where Woody Allen's father tells him that one day all this land will be yours, and it's that piece of sod with the little houses and village on it? And the deathbed scene where the herring king husband of Keaton says lying there what a pure wife she's been, but that just once, that sex just once would have been nice, and the guys standing behind her can't stop laughing, even the priest has laid her." John slapped his hands on the steering wheel, and when he got talking real fast, looking over at me the whole time, and laughing, he forgot he was driving, and I had to shout at him to miss the blue Mercedes heading toward us.

We stopped at the shed at the entrance to the parking lot and greeted the girl who checked the car stickers. She had blond hair and a nice smile. We had gotten there early enough so that we got a space near the old wooden ramps on either side of the wooden beach pavilion that had bathrooms in it and a hot dog, candy and soda stand at the front, facing the ocean; it was run by an old Tugboat Annie type who had fallen on bad times. John left his sandals in the car; he just wore them for driving, refusing to admit that the soles of your feet could burn off on the hot pavement of the parking lot or on the sand, especially the sand that was up by the dunes. He got the cooler out and the beach umbrella, with the metal frames of the low beach chairs hooked over the umbrella, and I carried the towels, his book and sunglasses and my satchel of *The New York Times*, a book, Block Out sun lotion, head bandannas, three dollars, and the car keys that John had just dropped in. We got to the top of the ramp and walked onto the deck of the beach pavilion, then stood looking left and right as we did every time. It was still early enough so that there was empty sand all around, but we knew the area around the lifeguard's chair would fill up soon with the teenagers and their radios. The noise they made was easy to avoid; what was not so easy was picking out the families or groups of singles that might have under one of their towels a paddleball set.

We always went left. Way, way down the beach to the left. This day the nice old gay man who owned the house we passed to get to our usual spot was out walking. He always nodded and smiled at us, and John said good morning. This morning he was alone. We had noticed his male houseguests were getting younger and younger, and I, at least, felt sad that he probably thought he had to keep in extra-good physical shape to get the younger ones. I still see him. He opens his house in the spring and closes it I guess a little after Thanksgiving. I've always wanted to say hi to him, or I guess really explain to him why John is no longer with me, why I'm there just with my little boy. He and John talked a few times, and John would come back saying what a nice guy he was, and I just wish I could get up the courage to say hello to him now. He seems to be alone now more often, often sitting on a chair on the deck of his house by himself. Have the young ones no use for him anymore? He smiles when he sees me and my son, and I get the feeling he would like to say hello as much as I would like to. I'm just too shy.

John set up the beach chairs, jabbed the steel shaft of the umbrella into the sand, twisting it down farther and farther until he was satisfied that no wind could blow it away. He sat down for maybe five minutes, telling me about the tennis that morning with Tony, about how Tony could be a really first-class player if he just had more confidence in himself. John was one of those people who was certainly always trying to improve his serve or his backhand but basically thought tennis was really a mental war, with confidence giving one a leading edge, and he just didn't understand why Tony, whom he admired so much, just didn't seem to have that extra push of self-confidence.

I told John not many people have that, that most of us are weakly trying to keep ourselves afloat.

Sometimes I felt I was an interpreter for John, as he was for me. He reported the optimist's side of life; I reported on the ways and actions of the pessimists. No, not really the pessimists, but the group of humans who find life a difficult business even under the happiest of circumstances. And I shouldn't have said optimists either; I meant the group of humans who find life a joy even under the unhappiest of circumstances. That's what I mean. I told John I could waffle back and forth, analyze and try to explain to myself so that I could understand the words and actions of the people I met and of myself, and John scratched his head—does her mind really turn over these little details? he wondered—and he said, well, it must work, because I had the best perception of people of anybody he'd ever known, and I said to him that so did he, we just got there in different ways.

"Now that we've got that settled," I told John, "how about you and me, um, er . . ."

"Jesus, Nini, here on the beach?"

I winked. "Or we could read our books. Up to you, Bunk." He rolled out of a beach chair and pulled my hand so I landed on top of him, gave me a kiss, and said, "God, I love you, Nini. Don't ever leave me, Little One." Then, "How about a swim?"

John jumped up and started to run to the water, and I yelled for him to take off his watch, which he always forgot to do unless I remembered just as he was about to dive under the first wave, and he came back to the chairs shaking his head, his eyes squinting at me in the sun, and handed me his watch, and said, "What a good girl you are, Nini."

Sometimes I thought we were the only two married people who never called each other dear, honey, sweetie, darling, whatever, we just used nicknames, the variety of which grew larger every year. But after seven summers and almost four years of marriage, Bunky and Nini had established permanency.

John was never as happy as when he was swimming in that blue ocean water. He was the first to admit that he was not a very good swimmer—not that he wasn't strong, but he splashed about a lot. And when he got hit by a wave he hadn't seen coming and was knocked over, he came up grinning. He was the first one in the water on Memorial Day weekend, and I saw him swim into October. That July morning he convinced me that I had to come in—"The water's glorious," he said—but then he said that even when there were gray high waves and it looked as if it was about to rain.

This morning he was right. It was one of those rare clear blue-water days, the waves were just the right size for easy rides in, and you could see your feet when the phosphorus cleared. The sand under the water was a steady, gradual slope into deeper water; there was no two-foot surprise of a drop-off so that you were standing with the water between your chest and waist one minute and the next minute you were way over your head because you had stepped off the shelf. No, he was right, that day was perfect. I gradually walked in, and when the water reached my waist and I couldn't stand the cold any longer I dove under a wave. John swam underwater around my legs, and had I not been pregnant he would probably have grabbed my bathing suit and pulled me under the water with him and then somehow swum under my legs so that he could raise me up high over his shoulders and then throw me backward into the water. Now, though, he just gave me a pinch to remind me of those times, and to say that as a prospective father he knew he'd better not be too rough with me. We swam up and down for about twenty minutes. A lot of the time I floated on my back thinking about the two of us and the baby we were going to have and watching the seagulls.

I got out first and wrapped a towel around myself. The year before I also would have dived into my satchel for matches and a cigarette. I quit in February when one of my favorite people at Nightingale was operated on for cancer and was told that she must stop smoking. I made a deal with her, I'd quit if she would, and told her that this was a big step for me, I hadn't even quit for John, although he'd made it clear to me that that would be the nicest present I could give him. Well, Betty was able to go without a cigarette for a month; I still hadn't had one and of course wouldn't have one now that I was pregnant, but I was surprised at the vivid memories of after-swim cigarettes. It is amazing how infertility or loneliness, when one is single, can make one feel one deserves a few vices, smoking, drinking.

I handed John back his watch, and we settled back to our books and some iced tea. Seven summers on these beaches. The same beach towels every summer, the same sheets no matter what house we were in, the sadness at finally throwing away a many-summers bathing suit with no elastic left in it, the above-the-knee cotton dresses that were no longer in fashion, how I used to have to cover myself with something called Nosekote because seven summers before there had been no sunscreen lotions, the summer we threw away the tube of Crest and bought some new blue stuff called Aim. When I first met John I still put my hair up in rollers; now I could blow it dry. Loss of favorite but now too threadbare or out-of-date clothing and upper Madison Avenue innovations, stores, restaurants. I don't like anything to change. I didn't like that new house going up on Dune Road, not just because it was ugly, but because it forced me to admit that one is never isolated from change, even in one's tiny protected sphere.

"John, listen to this." I read him a few lines about the Steering School in *The World According to Garp*. About three times that morning I had started to laugh out loud, and John would say, "What's so funny? Okay, okay, come on, tell me, read it to me." So by the time I got to the part where Garp bites the ear off that villainous dog Bonkers, John said he had to read the book for himself. Any character who bit a dog sounded great to him.

John that morning had Dickens' *Bleak House* on his lap. He and his friend Tony had decided that during their July vacations they were (1) going to play tennis every day and (2) read *Bleak House*. Tony was a partner in the corporate department at Milbank Tweed, and John, although in the tax department at his firm, had spent a good part of his eight years there on an estate on which work had begun in 1952 and still wasn't resolved, so he and Tony looked forward to a four-week submersion in the intricacies of the case of Jarndyce and Jarndyce. And the Dickens names: Dedlock, Smallweed, Chadband, Jellyby. John had on a pair of chrome-framed sunglasses that he called his Italian Via Veneto sunglasses—he knew they were awful and garish, but he loved them—and after I finished reading the cause of my most recent laughter, he put his sunglasses up on his head, slapped his hands down on his knees and said, "How about a walk, Nini?" It was about ten-fifteen.

We usually walked only as far as the pink house, a house that is attributed to Sanford White (we never knew, but we liked to think it was true), but that day we walked all the way down the beach to the Ocean Road beach. We passed a shingle house with a stone chimney; there were yellow umbrellas over the two tables on the deck, the deck chairs were royal blue, and a late-fiftyish couple walked out with their coffee mugs and sat on their deck. The wife finished her coffee and walked down the steps to the beach where we were walking. She looked like a gardener, even though the sand dunes around their house probably only sustained portulaca, but she was a woman with a schedule, and this was obviously her morning walk. She happily waved a goodbye to her husband, and he responded with a wave of his own and a smile, and went into the house with the breakfast dishes piled in his arms. Bet he was going to wash them or at least put them into the dishwasher, just bet that, he looked like he would.

We smiled as the woman passed us and went toward the beach we'd just come from. John began to do a little jogging; he was getting ahead of me. I put my hands on my hips, lifted my sunglasses and rested them on my head over a blue bandanna, and looking out at the ocean, the sun still low enough to glint on the surface of the water, I watched the waves break. This, I thought, was complete happiness. I was happy, my husband was happy. And then I had a thought, a terrible, ugly freakish thought as I looked upon the sea. I said to myself silently, "Enjoy this moment, Nancy. You'll never have another one like it, because John is going to die and you're going to be a widow."

I blinked my eyes and fast turned my head around to look for John in the distance. He waved his arms over his head; he was jogging backward, still looking at me, thought I had forgotten him, and he waved his hand for me to walk ahead and then to run and meet him. I ran a few steps and then theatrically patted my hand on my chest to give him the idea that I was out of breath. He walked toward me, and he would never, never know that I thought right then that I was going to lose him. God knew how. Probably in a car accident, or perhaps a plane accident if he had to go to Europe again, or there was talk

of another trip to Mexico. I wanted to kill my mind for
thinking the thought of his death. Why the hell, I wondered to myself, couldn't I enjoy each moment as it was
lived instead of unconsciously loading my mind with
doom? What an aberrant thought. That was all there was
to it. I gave John a kiss and we continued our walk, but I
could have killed myself for ruining it with that terrible
unsolicited thought.

That was our last week of vacation. A week later we
would be back at our desks. We started walking back to
our chairs and the beach umbrella, John's arm around my
shoulder, our feet walking at the edge of the breaking
waves. A two-engine propeller plane flew overhead, its
altitude far too low to be legal. John asked me if I could
feel the baby yet. I liked to think that the faint flutterings I
sometimes felt were the baby, but it was probably just my
stomach rumbling. We began to talk about names. John
said he'd like to name a boy after his father, Vincent, or
maybe use Vincent as a middle name. I said I'd like to
name him John. "Really, Nini?" "Sure." The girl's name
was easy. John said how about Katherine, and I agreed.
Or maybe Nancy, he added. No, I liked Katherine. Oh,
wait, I've got it, said John. Let's call a boy Rudy! Isn't that
awful? Rudy Rossi! I guess other couples have had funny,
private, pre-birth names for their children, and Rudy became ours. Instead of asking how I felt and how the baby
was, John would ask, "How's Rudy?"

After lunch we packed up and went home to read and
take naps, John complaining about how hot the sand and
the parking-lot pavement were under his bare feet; he
skipped on his toes as fast as he could to the car, trying to
stay on the white-painted lines of the parking spaces, and
as he unlocked the car the rush of hot vinyl upholstery air
hit his face. Towels went on the seats, and we rolled down
the windows and opened the side vents as fast as we

could. We decided to skip buying the corn that day. We would go out to dinner that night, maybe that Spanish place in Southampton, have a margarita and some sangria, they took American Express. Our American Express bill for July would be huge. John rarely carried any cash, and I had brought out maybe only two hundred dollars for the whole month. Everything else, from tennis balls to restaurants, went on American Express. Did I have some cash left? Yes. Well then why not go to a movie afterward?

I remember thinking after John died that we were so lucky to have had our time in July. It was different from other times out there, because for the first time we weren't sharing a house. Menus weren't planned with others, and I know I missed that at first. In the mornings we'd sometimes talk over the idea of inviting another couple over for dinner, but by the afternoon, having showered and lying on our bed, naked, with the sea breeze blowing through the curtains, having made love and now reading our books or just resting or talking, we'd decide that actually we'd rather just be with each other that evening. During the whole four weeks I think we went to friends once for dinner, and they and other friends came for dinner once at our house. Often I'd thought in the past that by surrounding ourselves with our friends, seeing them as much as three or four times a week, our marriage, the high level of camaraderie in our marriage, would be sustained, even increased. What we discovered that July was that we could share ourselves with each other as much and more and better than we had with our friends. We continued our more secluded life even when we returned to New York in August, and, of course, by the end of September there were no other people, much less friends, in our lives except for doctors.

Thinking about our last summer together has a painful

haze of unreality about it. I have a photograph of John
taken that July on the beach, and his eyes seem to stare
beyond the camera rather than looking toward it. What is
he thinking about? And another one of the two of us, our
backs to the camera, walking down the beach, John's arm
around my shoulder, his head bowed down to mine, talking to me so earnestly, this I do remember, that I was
going to be such a good mother, how very proud he was
of me, how much he needed me, that he loved me more
than anyone he'd ever known, and that I'd changed his
life, had made him happy. "Yeah, sure," he said, "this
partnership thing's on my mind, but if they don't make
me one, fuck 'em, I can always leave, and anyway, I've got
the Little One. What more could I ask for?" And he really
meant it.

In August we visited John's family in Utica. August is
one of the most beautiful months there, and with John's
brother's birthday being August 16, we had a happy reason to go there every summer. We both got out of work
early on an August Friday and by two o'clock were crossing the Tappan Zee Bridge to get onto the New York State
Thruway. And each time we crossed that bridge, each
time we drove up to Utica over the years, John would recall how much longer the drive used to take before the
thruway was built. John could repeat stories over and over
again about things that had happened to him, things he
remembered, and at the same spots on the thruway John
would retell the history of the Mohawk Valley and Mohawk River, and I would encourage him, prompting him
as we passed various landmarks, and asking him to tell me
again about the Hudson River painters he admired so
much, about the time he drove from New York to Utica,
before the 55-mile-an-hour speed limit, in three and a half
hours, about summer family excursions to Adirondack
lakes.

One of his favorites would begin when we got off the thruway in Utica and headed over the bridge into the city. John would start off by saying, "Nini, this bridge wasn't here when we came up here last." And I'd say, "Of course it was, it's been here for ages." And John would always reply, "They keep changing the roads here!" Once, when we drove to a movie theater in a nearby new shopping mall, he completely lost his sense of direction coming back and had us driving toward Syracuse, even though I kept telling him we were going in the wrong direction. He didn't believe me until he saw a sign which indicated we were a lot closer to Syracuse than to Utica. And he was incredulous. "Nini, how did you know we were going the wrong way? You didn't even grow up here!"

However, going over the bridge to downtown Utica meant John had at least ten blocks on Genesee Street to tell me about the time he was a paper boy. He'd point to various houses as we passed them and tell me about their inhabitants back in the '50s. He liked being a paper boy, liked being up early in the morning and having the responsibility and the independence of traveling on his bike. But he didn't like any of the residents who lived in the one apartment building on his route. There were mean old ladies in the building, he said, who demanded that he leave their papers outside their doors instead of in the downstairs lobby. There was no elevator in the building, and lugging the papers up the stairs took time and annoyed him, especially when a Christmas season passed and not one of the tenants gave him a tip.

But the glee in his voice and face would return as we passed buildings and streets with happier memories. "That's where I learned to ride a bike. There's the house I grew up in—it's in such bad shape now; you should have seen it the way my mother kept it, beautiful!—and there's the Kimball Street School, my elementary school! I was in

a parochial school at first, during nursery school and kindergarten, but I hated it. My grandmother, though, was a
very important member of the Catholic church in this par-
ish, and I always had the feeling I had to be the best and
never do anything wrong, because if I got into trouble, I'd
get it not only from the sisters but from my grandmother,
too."

A few blocks after we turned left onto the parkway,
a wide tree-lined boulevard, John would point out the
statue of Christopher Columbus. "It's dedicated to my
grandfather, you know." John was very proud of that. His
grandfather had gotten his medical degree in Italy and had
decided to come to America. John wasn't sure how, but
his grandfather had heard that Utica had a large Italian
population and that he would be happy there. The difference in climates must have appalled him that first winter.
He settled there, though, and became the first Italian surgeon in Utica and the first Italian doctor allowed operating
privileges at not only the Catholic hospitals but at the Prot-
estant ones as well. He married a pretty, tiny girl, Adelina
Tetti, who had grown up in Baltimore and now was a
teacher in Utica. She was one of five sisters, all of whom
became adoring aunts when her daughter and son were
born, John's aunt and father. Along with Dr. Rossi's success as a doctor in the community came a house he bought
on Rutger Street for his family. It is now the headquarters
of a social-service program there, but one can still see its
former opulence in its exterior Victorian ornamentation.
John would drive me past it and tell me it was huge inside
as well and how he remembered Sunday dinners and
Christmases there.

Dr. Rossi's two children went to the only private school
in Utica, and his son Vincent, John's father, then went to
Harvard and, deciding he had heard enough gory details
about medicine from his father at the dinner table, con-

tinued at Harvard Law School, where he met a beautiful fairy princess of a girl who lived in Boston and was a nurse. For reasons I've never been able to understand, Dr. Rossi and his wife did not want their son to marry her, perhaps because she was not Italian but rather half Irish and half Swedish, or perhaps they had someone else in mind for him back home in Utica. Fortunately Vincent didn't listen to them, and he married Esther Anderson in 1943. After his service in the war as an Air Force radar officer, he and Esther moved to Utica, where he started his law practice and where Esther and her mother-in-law formed an uneasy truce made easier, surely, by the presence of Esther and Vincent's first child, their toddler son, John, who was born in 1945, and who was then followed by Vincent Jr. in 1947, Mary Ellen in 1951, and Patricia in 1956.

John once told me, with a grin on his face, that his father would tell him that he could be a doctor, a lawyer or a bum when he grew up. Was his father serious? I asked. Oh, yes. John, like his father, hated the thought of medicine, although he was brilliant at chemistry and physics, and decided to follow his father into law. For one thing he liked to talk, and he knew he'd have the opportunity to talk as much as he wanted as a lawyer, and he had some hope of getting into politics. John did "C" work in college at Colgate University—he wasn't accepted at Harvard or later on at Harvard Law—and with his father's help, he was accepted by Cornell Law School. Did "C" work there, too, but he took a tax course with a professor who knew his father and who encouraged him and told him he had a talent for tax work, so that when interview time came and the big New York firms sent representatives to the campus, the tax professor suggested that John have an interview with the people from Kelley Drye, and he would recommend him to the partners he knew there.

John often said that were he in college now, he never would have gotten into such a good law school, and that not being anywhere near the top of his law school class, he certainly would not have been offered the job at Kelley Drye. John by that time was one of the two youngest members of Kelley Drye's applicant review committee and was an interviewer himself at law schools. That August, just after we returned from Utica, he interviewed applicants for two days up at Columbia Law School, and his favorite one was a young man who told John with a straight face that ever since he'd been a child his goal had been to become a lawyer with Kelley Drye. ("Jesus, Nini, can you believe that guy actually *said* that?") John found it unnerving to turn down many of the applicants whose grades and rank in class numbers were much higher than his had been. "Boy," he'd say, "I got in just under the wire. No big firm would look at me today." His parents had been hoping that after law school he would return to Utica and join his father's firm, but they accepted his desire to try working for a big New York City firm first and see how well he did there.

Marrying into the Rossi family showed me how much fun it is to be a member of a big family, what it's like to sit at a dining-room table with all the leaves in it. In addition to John's parents, there'd be his brother, sometimes with a girlfriend, and both sisters, sometimes with their boyfriends, and John's father's sister, Aunt Linuccia, who was a widow and who, having no children of her own, was pleased to be such an important part of her nephews' and nieces' lives. She often came down to New York on bus trips with friends of hers to go to Broadway shows, and John and I would meet her before the show began for lunch or afterward for dinner. And as John and I got out of the car, his mother was soon there at the kitchen door, beaming at John and then coming out to greet us and to tell us how well we both looked, tanned from our time at the beach.

John glowed that weekend. He told his father about reading *Bleak House*, he told him it looked as if he'd be doing more traveling for the firm, that a trip to Mexico City was coming up in September, and there was talk with his mother and father about the baby-to-be; Aunt Linuccia had already started knitting blankets for the baby's carriage and crib. We had a family dinner at home on Friday night, and on Saturday John's father said there was a restaurant he'd like to take us to in the country. Vincent was off to see his girlfriend that weekend, and Mary Ellen was down at Cooperstown with her friends, so early Saturday evening, John and I and his parents, his sister Patricia and Aunt Linuccia got into the Mercedes to drive to the place.

It wasn't far out of Utica, as the roads became smaller, more rural, more hilly, that I began to feel sick. I'd never been carsick before, but the motion of the car, up and down the hills, was making me sick. I couldn't take my mind off it, and I panicked. Oh, God, I thought, I'm going to lose this baby right here. The car continued on the winding roads, and I felt as if I were going to cry. The car ride was getting worse, it was like a rollercoaster, and I felt that except for John, who kept looking over his shoulder at me with a worried expression from the passenger seat up front next to his father, who was driving, nobody cared that I was going to throw up. John told his father he was going to take over the driving, and he did his best to make the drive not quite as bumpy. We'd been driving for forty minutes or so, and my head was spinning, and when we at last reached the restaurant, John's sister said I looked sick. I certainly felt sick, and John followed me up a path, where I did get sick and began to cry.

I was a child. Through my tears I told him that nothing must happen to this baby, that I must get home. I just wanted to get into bed. I held him so tightly. I think now that had I known this was the last time we would be going out to dinner as a family together, I would have shaped up, snapped out of it, and behaved like an adult. As it was, John returned to his parents and told them we had to drive home. Later when I was in my bed upstairs, his mother brought me some tea and soup and crackers. I was very embarrassed, but my mother-in-law told me not to worry, that being pregnant was not easy, she knew, having had more than one miscarriage of her own.

A couple of weeks later John was to be the best man at the wedding of his good college friend Mike Rubenstein. I decided not to risk being sick on a plane, so John flew to Rochester by himself. He called me from his motel room frequently, said he wasn't feeling too great, maybe it was the heat, but all he wanted to do was sit inside with the air conditioner, and worst of all the tuxedo he had to wear for the wedding was awfully tight around the waist. He said he was going to stay inside and watch television until it was time for him to get ready for the wedding.

This was not like him, and I worried. John would normally be outside jogging, no matter how hot it was. He flew back the next day, and I wonder now if maybe even then he had started to look a little different. At the beach the next weekend he complained about how he looked in a bathing suit. His stomach did seem to be sticking out more than it had the week before. I teased him that he must have eaten everything at the wedding reception himself.

Before Labor Day weekend he made an appointment for a checkup: his back was bothering him, too. Maybe he'd hurt it playing tennis; anyway, we both agreed that he should check it out with the doctor. He had some X-rays, which seemed to show nothing, but the pain in his back did not go away. He did stretching exercises, which seemed to make him feel better, and he was to see the doctor again after Labor Day weekend.

John put down *Garp*. We were still on the beach in the late afternoon, watching the seagulls and terns and sandpipers take over the beach as the people left. Soon we would go and take showers at home and get ready to go out for dinner. I asked him how he was enjoying *Garp*—a little bit easier going than *Bleak House*, right? He put his sunglasses on top of his head, and as he sat in his beach chair, he looked out at the ocean, and then looked down at the book in his lap and then over to me.

"I'm not going to finish this, Nini. I don't like it."

"Really? Why?"

"It's not as funny as I thought it was going to be, and"—John was so good at predicting the endings of movies, the murderer in a mystery—"Garp's going to die, isn't he?"

I reached over and took the book out of his hands. "How far did you get?" He showed me: he wasn't even halfway through. And I said, "Well . . ."

"I knew it," John said. "That guy's my age, and he's going to die."

"But Bunky, people do die in books; that's no reason not to finish it."

"Well, I can't help it. It's depressing. Be a good girl and take it back to the library," and he got up and started running down the beach.

Hmmm, no use talking him out of it, I thought, and I told myself to drop it, not to mention it when he returned, and put the book into the beach bag.

I remembered this incident not too long ago and shivered. John couldn't have known he was going to die then, back in July, at the beach, could he?

CHAPTER FOUR

On Labor Day weekend John and I had one of our very infrequent quarrels. He was angry with me for inviting our friends Rodd and Janet for the weekend. "I just wanted to be alone with you, Little One."

"Bunky, I'm sorry, I made a mistake, I thought you would be pleased, thought we could play a little bridge, cook some good dinners . . ."

"Well, I'm not. Sure, I like them. I just wanted to be with you this weekend. Shit."

"Oh, come on, John, this isn't like you. Usually you like having company."

"Not this weekend."

"I am sorry, Bunky, truly. But there's not much I can do

about it now. They're on their way out here. Come on, buck up, Uncle Buckle, we'll have fun."

"I suppose so."

Oh, I felt awful. I'd thought we had talked about having them out for that weekend, but I should have asked John more recently, and I hadn't, I just went ahead and invited them. Later on when he came down from taking a shower, I apologized, saying I should have checked with him before I invited them. "Don't worry about it, Nini. I'm sorry I blew up. You're right, we'll have fun, and of course I'm looking forward to seeing them. Don't worry, Little One."

The next day on the beach, I was sitting under the umbrella with Rudd and Janet; they had bought some land in Amagansett and we were talking about the house they wanted to have built on it someday. They had been talking to a few architects. I asked Janet if she had heard any good gossip recently from her voice teacher about the opera world. Oh, yes, Janet laughed—oh, I wish I could describe her laugh, it sounds like bells and clear splashing water falling over pebbles in a river—and she told me that Tenor X was having an affair with Soprano Y and, of course, both were married to others, and they thought no one knew but, of course, everyone in the opera world did know. Janet grew up outside of Portland, got a master's degree in library science, worked in the Harvard Law School library and then decided to go to law school herself. Her law school class at Harvard gave John and me most of our friends, and many of them started their careers at Kelley Drye as well. Along with her legal work, Janet also continued to take voice lessons.

There was nothing more lovely in the old Bayberries house than to hear her practicing at the piano on a quiet summer afternoon. And when John and I were planning our wedding, we asked her if she would sing. We agreed on "Panis Angelicus," and my parents had a tape machine next to them to record the service; the only thing you can really hear is her clear voice. I remember asking her in my state of numbness after John died if she would sing it again at his memorial service. I somehow wanted to wrap up our marriage that way, but of course I knew she wouldn't be able to do it and probably thought I was a little crazy even to ask her. Instead a man from the church's own choir sang it. She apologized, saying she was sorry, but that—and she started to cry—John meant so much to all of us, and she didn't think she could handle it, it would be too sad for her.

John had, in fact, introduced Rodd and Janet to each other. Rodd was a friend he'd met during his Army Reserve days. They both had to go up to the Bronx for their weekend meetings and went together for the two weeks of summer camp each year. One of my most treasured letters of those that arrived after John died was from Rodd, and he remembered a time when I called John at summer camp, and Rodd was with him, and he said John's face lighted up with the biggest smile when I told him I'd found an apartment for us to live in together. Rodd and John played bridge often, and one evening John brought Janet to be his partner. That was the first time they met, and they were married six months after we were.

Rodd also was a member of the Opera Club and had helped John join, and for the past year he'd been trying to convince John to join the University Club, since they knew him so well there anyway. In fact, he and David Clark used to laugh that the club would have to establish "the John Rossi Rule," meaning that members were restricted in the number of times they could bring a guest to play squash, except, it seemed, for John Rossi, because he knew enough people who were members that he was there sometimes more than once a week, and David and Rodd joked that the rules committee had started to notice.

John had said, sure, he'd love to join, "the Little One and I just have to rob a gas station for the money, that's all." But then he became serious and thought that after the first of the year, after the baby was born, and hoping that maybe he'd be a partner at Kelley Drye beginning then, yes, he would like to be nominated for membership.

A couple of weeks after John died, Rodd took me there for dinner. Janet was in Chicago for a convention, and he, like others, wanted to get me out, cheer me up. We had a drink first in the green lounge and then went up to the seventh floor to the main dining room for dinner. It is a beautiful wood-paneled room with terrifically high ceilings and large windows. I told Rodd it reminded me of Columbia, and he said, yes, Low Library, the reading room. Same McKim Mead White architects. I was jealous of all the handsome young men in the room—John should have been one of them. Gruesomely I could easily picture each with cancer and what it would do to their faces and bodies.

As we left, Rodd asked if I would like to see the library; he wanted to show it to me. We got on the elevator, and were about to step off at the library floor, but I got only a peek as the elevator doors opened and an elderly man came into the elevator. I made a step forward to pass him, and he boomed out, "Where are you going?" I quickly stepped back inside the elevator, as did Rodd. "Don't you know," he said to Rodd, glaring, "that ladies are not allowed on this floor?" Rodd, of course, had known, but he had probably thought, hell, it's a quiet January night, who's going to notice? It was funny in a way, me only three weeks away from delivering the baby, my stomach sticking out in front of me, and Rodd trying to cheer me up by giving me an evening out, and here was this only-go-by-the-rulebook rude old man treating us like very,

very naughty children. It was embarrassing at the time, but now I can laugh about it.

John had gotten up while Janet was talking, gotten up very abruptly, and started running down the beach. The three of us looked at each other and shrugged our shoulders.

"Is John feeling okay?" Rodd asked.

"Oh, yeah," I replied, "he's fine."

But in the distance we could see him doing jumping jacks, and he looked as if he were on fire, very agitated, very nervous. The whole weekend he was like that: rude, abrupt, not able to sit still, and if he was not running or doing jumping jacks, he was rotating his arms above his head and rubbing his back.

Rodd and Janet wondered if John was becoming nervous about the partnership decisions to be made at the end of the month. "No," I said, "I don't think so." He had never been nervous about it before. He certainly had put in long hours and wanted that achievement more than anything, but he had always had a sensible, humorous perspective about the procedure. Now I was not so sure. His behavior was making me nervous, and I was frightened.

The next weekend we stayed in the city. We went for a walk in the park on Saturday morning, but John tired after not even ten minutes, and we had to sit down on a bench. He had been seeing his doctor and other specialists all week. The X-rays showed nothing. Even he was appalled that he had to rest on the bench. "I don't know what's the matter with me, Little One. I'm so tired all the time. You know that's not like me."

"You going back to Dr. Lisio next week?" I asked.

"Yeah, I guess I'll see him when he gets the report back from the lab."

I explained to John about his birthday coming up that week. "I decided to combine your birthday and partnership present—"

"Partnership present?"

"Sure, they're going to make you a partner."

"Let's wait until the returns are in."

"Well, anyway, I've bought you something that I'm going to give you when they make the announcement."

In late August I had gone to two luggage and leather stores, Mark Cross and T. Anthony, and priced attaché cases. John's old one, he had complained, was falling apart, the locks didn't work anymore, it wasn't big enough to hold all the papers he had to take when he was traveling, and he wanted one with a combination lock. Maybe, he said, he'd spring for one next year. Well, I spent a whole afternoon looking at them and was shocked at how expensive they were, but they were beautifully made. A nice man at Mark Cross finally helped me choose the right one. It was lovely, and I told the salesman to go ahead and have John's initials put on it. I just knew he was going to be so pleased with it and with me for going ahead and getting him something he really wanted.

"So," I asked him, "what would you like to do on your birthday? Would you like to go out for dinner or stay home and have me cook something?"

"Oh, that would be fine, Nini. Let's stay home, just the two of us."

"You want me to make the veal with that mustard sauce?"

"Yeah, that would be good."

"And I'll bake some kind of cake."

"Sounds great, Little One."

"You ready to leave here?" I asked. "You want to keep walking or head back home?"

"I think . . . I think we'd better head home, Nini. Maybe I'll check out the Yankee game on television."

John's birthday was on Wednesday, September 6. He was thirty-three years old. For most of the year we were three years apart, but during the time between his birthday and mine in January we were four years apart. I wouldn't be thirty until January 31. Thirty-three seemed very old to me that fall; John had always been the older and wiser partner, and I tried to imagine myself being thirty-three and I couldn't. This winter when I did turn thirty-three, I realized how very young it is, that I'm not measurably wiser, just older, and that it is only the title of widow that makes me feel truly old, that I have lived out of sequence somehow. That now I should be a mother with a young son and a husband, planning more children, thinking about getting a bigger apartment as the family grows, going to the zoo as a whole family, but instead I am a mother of a young son and am also a widow. It shouldn't have happened until I was in my seventies, I think. And what do I have in common with widows in their sixties and seventies? Not much.

And I also no longer have much in common with women my own age, with the exception of talking about our young children. They begin talking about entertaining clients, late hours at the office, promotions, job changes, restaurants, the Opera Club, oh, and vacations are the worst, "Oh, we just had to get away from the kids for a while, so they stayed with their grandparents, and we flew down to Bermuda, stayed at a lovely old inn in Connecticut for the weekend, decided to see what Block Island looked like in the winter, went skiing in Colorado." I can't listen; I don't know what they're talking about, and at those times I realize I do, grudgingly, have more in common with widows. It's just that I'm not sure what group I belong to, because actually I don't belong to either one. So this winter when I turned thirty-three, it was a shock to realize that very, very soon I will have been alive longer than John, that from now on I will be older than he was when he died, and that twenty years from now I'll still be thinking of him at thirty-three when I am fifty-three, and it'll be like thinking about a young man who by then is a stranger to me.

When he came home from work that day I could tell he wasn't feeling well, and he looked tired. We sat down for the dinner I had cooked, and he barely picked at it. He was appreciative, but he didn't have anything to say and seemed annoyed when I tried to keep the conversation, any conversation, alive. Even the elaborate Julia Child cake I'd worked on that afternoon didn't appeal to him. He apologized, saying he didn't know why, but he just wasn't hungry, and a few moments later he quickly left the dinner table and went back to our bedroom and read. It seemed he wouldn't talk to me. I kept asking him what was wrong, and he just got mad. I went out to the kitchen to do the dishes, and I was scared; he had never treated me like that before. I worried that he didn't want the baby, didn't want me. This was the first birthday night of his since I'd met him in 1972 that we didn't make love.

But two nights later our eyes locked together, and together we looked down at his bulging stomach as we lay in bed, and no one now needed to tell us why we were scared. He had only his shorts on and his stomach was bulging, huge, the blue veins showing beneath the thin translucence of his skin. I never knew there were so many veins and arteries over our stomachs. And that's what scared me.

And I said, "John, what is this? What's wrong?" and pointed to those veins.

And he answered, "I don't know, Nini." His face was as full of fear as mine.

And I said, "You've got to go back to Dr. Lisio."

John said, "I've got an appointment in a few days."

And me: "No, you must go before then—tomorrow!"

John laughed and said Kathy Davis, Tom's wife—Tom, the fellow who had the office next door to him in the tax department—that Kathy said maybe his large stomach was a "sympathetic pregnancy." John even got up off the bed and found my Freud book in the bookcase to look it up. Maybe it was psychological, he said.

"Now, Nini, it's all right."

"But, John, I've never seen anything like this, these veins." And I thought of my own stomach and the way it looked at the beginning of my sixth month of pregnancy. It was big, but there were no veins showing through. John told me he was not going to Mexico for the firm as planned the next week. He had asked Dr. Lisio about it and he had agreed and offered to write a note. "I just don't think I can do it, Nini. I'm too tired. I'm afraid if I go down there, I'll get much worse and I'll be so far away from home, from Dr. Lisio and from you." And as I write this it sinks in that what he was afraid of was dying there.

September had always been such a happy month for us, John's birthday and on the 14th our wedding anniversary. Everything was different about that September. John went again to the X-ray lab and had a GI series. Results negative, colon was clear. Every test was negative, so what was going on? What was wrong with him? He was losing more and more weight, his stomach was getting larger, his back hurt, and nobody knew what was wrong with him. By Thursday the 14th, John said in the morning he couldn't go to work, he felt too sick, too weak. It was the first sick day he had had from Kelley Drye in all the eight years he had worked there. How I would nag him when he would insist on going to the office with the flu and a high fever and tell him that a day in bed would do wonders for him and his cold! Only on weekends would he succumb to nurse care in bed when he had the flu, not on a weekday.

He felt terrible about missing the Mexico trip. He was more withdrawn than ever on our anniversary, and I think he was glad to see me go off to work in the morning. What an anniversary. I felt so lonely, and he didn't want my help, didn't want me around, didn't want to talk to me. On my way home that afternoon I bought some flowers, for him and for me, to cheer us up, but when I walked into the apartment, the first thing I saw was a vase full of red roses with a card from him to me for our anniversary, our fourth anniversary. John was in our bedroom asleep.

How unlike our first anniversary, I thought, when we were at the beach at Bayberries, and John was so excited because he'd gone into East Hampton to order red carnations to be delivered to the house. I was so surprised when the florist's truck came up the driveway, and John was half skipping and jumping around me because he was so pleased with his surprise. His college friend Mike Rubenstein and his girlfriend were with us for the weekend, along with our friend Diane, one of John's best friends in the firm; she and John worked together in the tax department. Everyone gathered around and looked at me as I sat down on the lawn and opened the long white florist box, and inside there was a card, and on it John had written, "To the most wonderful wife in the world." Bless Mike Rubenstein. He had his camera and took a picture of me opening the box with John standing next to me looking down at me. And later that evening he took another picture of John, all dressed up in his white linen pants, blue shirt with Liberty-print tie, and yellow linen jacket, opening a bottle of champagne, and me sitting in one of the old faded, chintz-covered chairs with a glass of champagne in my hand, wearing that pleated cranberry cotton dress John liked so much.

That night three years later I thanked him for the flowers, gave him a kiss, no, he really wasn't hungry, no, there was nothing I could get him, and I brought him in a silly anniversary card I'd bought that day, brought it in to him as he was lying on our bed reading. Part of it said, "Please overlook the 'new leaves' that I talk about but seldom turn, please overlook my temper and the foolish things I do, but don't you dare overlook just how much I love you." And then I wrote, "You're more important to me than anyone or anything in the world. I love you!!" John read it and laughed. "Yes, Nini, you have been annoying recently—you really should try to control your temper better."

And he was not joking. I thought he was at first because we so rarely fought or got angry, but he meant it. I nodded my head and said, "I guess I didn't realize, John. I'm sorry, I'll be better."

That made him smile his old, dear smile at me, and he said, "I know, Little One, I know." He was lying there in his bathrobe as he said that, looking ashen. Thank God he had another appointment with Dr. Lisio the next day, I thought.

We went together to Dr. Lisio's office around ten or eleven the next morning. The X-rays and tests done over the past two weeks still appeared to show nothing, or else Dr. Lisio was not talking. We were confused and frightened as we went into his office together. John's appearance was changing daily, thinner and thinner, the weight shedding off him except for his stomach. Even Dr. Lisio, who had seen John earlier in the week, was shocked. He talked to us for a while and then went into the examining room with John. I sat in the chair next to his desk, the baby rumbling around inside, and prayed.

Dr. Lisio came out, and while John stayed in the examining room getting dressed he began to talk to me. He was making arrangements for John to be admitted to Columbia-Presbyterian right away. We were to go home and pack pajamas and toothbrush and stuff and from there get a cab up to the medical center and check in at Harkness Pavilion; they would be expecting John.

"What's wrong with him?" I asked.

"I don't know, Nance, we don't know, but I don't like the way he looks at all, and I want to do some tests on him up there, tests we can only do in the hospital. He looks totally different from when I saw him on Monday. I don't like it." And then I think he said, as I try to recall our talk together, "It's happening so fast."

He asked me how John's spirits were, had his mood changed at all.

"Has it ever," I told him. "I don't know him anymore, he's changed completely, and that's what scares me, that and his stomach. I don't understand why he's changed. He doesn't want to talk to me anymore, doesn't even want me in the same room with him, he avoids me." I wondered since Dr. Lisio was asking me these questions if maybe John was having a nervous breakdown.

"He's up for partnership at his law firm, right?" Dr. Lisio asked. "Maybe that has something to do with it—it's got to be on his mind."

"No, it's not just that, I wish it were. He's just different."

"Well," Dr. Lisio said, "I'm sure everything's going to be all right. You just get him home, pack a bag for him, and get him up to Harkness. That's where he belongs now."

John opened the door and stepped out, adjusting his tie around his neck, and I saw for the first time how big his shirt was on him, that the collar was far too big. As he sat down in the chair next to mine, Dr. Lisio called the hospital, made the arrangements for John's admittance, and told us he would see us later up there.

Both John and I had been going to Dr. Lisio, he since he started working in New York and I since our marriage. He also treated many of our friends. We trusted him, and John and I always had great Lisio stories to tell after either of us had gone to him for a checkup. One time he told John that he was perfectly fine but that he could probably lose five or ten pounds. John told him that he played tennis and squash and ran, that he got a lot of exercise, that he was always trying to get those extra pounds off, that he even walked to and from work, but that they just wouldn't come off. "And what, Doctor, do you do for exercise?" John asked. "What do you recommend?"

And Dr. Lisio, John told me, said, "Exercise? Exercise? Never do it. Don't have the time."

That story became part of John's repertoire. Once I came back and told John that Lisio was better than any psychiatrist I'd ever seen, that he asked very moving questions about how I was, how my marriage was going, how my spouse was, and then would launch into the joys of having children and say, "You, Nancy, really must have a child before you're thirty; it's more risky every year after that." He knew of my infertility, of course, and reassured me that something would happen. "I think, John," I said, "that Lisio may wish he'd gone into psychiatry."

Even though John was so weak we decided to walk home from 79th Street and Park Avenue. I asked him if maybe he would rather take a taxi. No, he wanted to walk. It would be the last time I saw him walk on Park Avenue. We got home, and John took off his jacket. He said he was so hot, and he sat down on the couch, his legs stretched out straight in front of him, one hand holding his back, his stomach jutting out in front of him, and he closed his eyes. I went back into our room and packed his bag.

Should I pack more than one pair of pajamas, I don't know, well I guess I should, okay, there're the blue ones and the yellow ones. Oh, yes, toothbrush, toothpaste. Yeah, and shaving stuff, a deodorant, anything else? Might want a book, I'll pack a mystery, one of the ones Diane left us. I went through Diane's stack of paperback mysteries, her solution for fear of flying in airplanes. Okay, that was it. Surely it would be a short, quick hospital stay, and they would say he had an ulcer or something. John meanwhile had come into the room and watched me pack as he sat on the bed, staring ahead, looking at nothing, looking exhausted. We got into the elevator, I carried his bag, then he took it from me as we walked through the lobby. Our doorman, Raymond, asked us where we were going. "To the hospital," John said. "Have to go in for some tests. I'll see you soon, Raymond."

We got into a cab and made the journey across 97th Street, through the park and over to the West Side Highway on which John had accompanied me so many times, for the two surgeries, for the infertility appointments with Uscher, and now I was taking him. The cab driver was not sure how to get there, and we told him exactly what exit to take—we always went up to the George Washington Bridge exit now that we had figured out that that way was faster and easier than getting off the drive at 152nd Street. At Harkness John was quickly seated in a wheelchair and taken upstairs while I filled out the admittance forms. As he was wheeled into the elevator, his eyes and mine locked for seconds, fully comprehending that although nobody had yet said anything to us, this was more serious than we had thought. The elevator doors closed and I returned to the paperwork.

I finished an hour later, I'd given them all the Blue Cross/Blue Shield information. I went into a phone booth and called my mother. "Yes," I said steadily, "Lisio's put

John in for some tests. Yes, I'm up at Harkness now. Yes, I'll call you later. Yes, it is a surprise." My mother was speechless: John in the hospital? I then went upstairs to John's room. He was in his pajamas in bed and a nurse was taking his temperature, blood pressure. He looked more comfortable than I had seen him in the past couple of weeks. As I looked up at the big color television suspended from the ceiling, I thought, Thank God, thank God John's Yankees have a good chance to reach the playoffs. He'll be able to watch the games.

We talked about calling his family. He told me we couldn't, that they would just worry. They knew John hadn't been feeling well, and they knew about his stomach. I told John it wasn't fair not to call them. He finally agreed, and we called them from the room. My mother-in-law told me later she knew right then that it was cancer; in fact, we told Lisio later that she thought that, and he asked John and me, "She said that to you?" I think now that maybe he had told them way before he wanted to break it to us.

The next ten days were agony for John as dozens of medical tests were performed, many quite painful. The worst was the arteriogram—they shot dye up his legs, which went through his system, and then they X-rayed him for long, agonizing minutes as he lay on a steel table. A day later we were told it had to be done again; the pictures hadn't come out. John almost cried at that news. "You don't know how much it hurts, Nini." All other tests came back negative for ten full days. It was worse than being told the truth, which they must have known by then. And it was worse for us. We talked and talked about what "it" could be. Had he wrenched his back playing tennis? That would be easy; that would explain the pain in his back. But why was his stomach so large? Why was he losing weight? How could John and I have been so naive?

Finally they told us they had found a tumor. Strangely, neither John nor I fell apart at this news. It was something definite. They held out their scrubbed, soft surgeon's hands to us in hope: it might be benign.

Meanwhile life at home had stopped. I didn't go in to school anymore, maybe a day here and there, but soon I would take a leave of absence. To save on cab money, my mother picked me up in the car after work. Soon she, too, would take a leave of absence so that she could drive me back and forth and stay with me in the apartment. Our cat sat in my lap every night. The phone never stopped ringing. How was John? Any news? No. I had my monthly checkup with Dr. Uscher. "They say the tumor is in the apron of the intestine," I told him. Then a few days later I spotted him early one Sunday morning going into the elevator in Harkness; seeing me he came out and we walked back into Presbyterian and took one of the hospital-bed-size elevators up. I told him everything, the results of the operation, everything, and he walked me through the hallways to Harkness and gestured for me to follow him into a small consulting room on John's floor.

We sat on a couch together and he asked me, "Are you all right?"

"Yes," I answered, "I'm okay. I don't believe it, but I'm okay."

"You sure?" he asked. I bit my lip and nodded my head and started to cry and nodded more furiously, trying to stop crying, "Yes, I'm okay."

He put his arms around me. There was nothing to say.

John was operated on on Tuesday, September 26, a day I will never forget. I arrived at the hospital at six in the morning. I knew from past experience when I was being operated on that a husband or wife would be let in at that early hour the day of an operation. I sat on the edge of John's bed with him and told him how much courage his

being with me before my operations gave me and that I
wanted to do the same for him. I advised him with a laugh
to keep some spit in his mouth because I was sure they
were going to give him the same floating tranquilizer, the
one that makes your mouth go dry before they finally
knock you out with the general. He laughed and thanked
me for the tip. He told me that Dr. Wiedel, the surgeon,
had wanted to see me yesterday and was disappointed I
had already left for the day when he came to John's room
around eight in the evening. John told me how much I
would like him. "He's very special, Nini, he's a real gentleman." I heard later that his nickname at the hospital
was "The Prince." Funny. That's how a lot of the people
in John's law firm referred to him, especially Diane—"The
Prince."

When John was moved to the stretcher, I gripped his
hand and kissed his cheek, "Everything's going to be all
right, Bunky, don't worry, and I'll be here waiting for you
when you return." Wiedel had told him he would probably be in the operating room for three or four hours.

The day before I had gone to a knitting and needlepoint
store called 2 Needles and a nice woman there had helped
me choose a daffodil pillow needlepoint design and had
gotten me started on the wool for the stems. I told her,
blurted out really, that it would be something for me to do
while my husband was being operated on, that a woman
at Nightingale had suggested it would help take my mind
off the time. She asked me what he was being operated on
for. Cancer, I told her. She looked at my pregnant stomach
and was stricken. She wished me luck.

I waved to John as he was wheeled out of the room, and
he waved back. The door began to close very slowly, and
there was a nurse who had stayed behind, and as I saw
John's sheet-covered feet disappear down the hall, she
said to me, "It's all right to cry." I turned quickly toward

her, angry, and shook my head, gesturing with my hand to the door still not fully closed. What I couldn't get out of my mouth was that I did not want John to hear me cry, but she was too fast, too eager to comfort, maybe she even knew this was a hopeless case, and she rushed over and put a hand on my shoulder and said again that I could cry, and a noise rose in my throat from animal depths and out heaved a cry. A cry for mercy, a cry to get her the hell out of the room, a cry I was terrified John had heard as he was being rolled into the large elevator. I had wanted him to go up to that operating room with my strength and confidence, not with the sound of my wail in his ears. I hated this nurse for interfering in our privacy. Remarkably and fortunately it was a rare instance of hospital stupidity that occurred during John's hospitalizations.

After she left I sat down in a chair by the window that had a footrest and got out my needlepoint. It felt good to get my feet up—they were starting to hurt, maybe because of the pregnancy, I don't know. I thought back over the past ten days. Every day I had brought things that John wanted from home along with the books that were arriving daily from friends and from people at the law firm, *Fools Die, Metropolitan Life,* which Rodd and Janet said in the note they wrote inside the cover should have been called "City Life," as that was one of John's favorite expressions—in fact, John's reaction to being in the hospital had almost also been "City life, Nini."

Right after John was admitted on September 15, we reached his parents, who came down as soon as they could and stayed with Esther's sister and husband, Aunt Helen and Uncle Jack, in Croton. And that's when I fell apart. I couldn't understand why they were looking at everything from the gloomiest point of view, why she was certain it was cancer, and John and I saying to each other that surely the doctors would have *told* us if that was the case. John wanted them to go back to Utica. Of course they couldn't, he was their son, their first child. And then I did something awful. The day before the operation, when his mother and I were sitting in John's room while he was walking in the hall with his father, she told me about the births of her children and how when Patricia, the youngest, was born there was a lesbian anesthesiologist who withheld longer than necessary, Esther said, the spinal and any other painkillers that were used in '56, just to frighten her. I'd been talking to her about how I was not going to try to gut out the delivery, that if the doctor thought I should be given something, I'd take it, which she thought was sensible. She still knew a lot about medicine from her nursing days and kept up with recent developments, but I couldn't understand why she was telling me this very scary story about the lesbian anesthesiologist. I tried to laugh. No, I thought, nobody here in this hospital would behave that way. And I heard Esther say, "I was pretty and young and she just had it in for me." Why was she telling me this?

That evening I called John's father in Croton and told him I did not want her or him at the hospital the next day, the day of John's operation, and I said to him, "You've known me a long time, Dad, you know I don't gossip, but I don't know what Ma was trying to do to me today, scaring me with this story, I don't understand it. I know everything will go smoothly with the pregnancy and the delivery, but I cannot be in the same room with her tomorrow. Tomorrow is something that John and I have to go through alone together."

Could they, he asked, at least sit downstairs in the Harkness lobby? I even said no to that, that they were not to be in the building at all. "I understand, kid, I understand," he said.

"We'll have the doctors call you as soon as they know

anything," I said. It's probably incomprehensible now to anyone why I did such a cruel, selfish thing. I suppose there was some kind of suppressed, unconscious fight going on between me and Esther for John, and I felt I had to hang on to him, to my title of wife, instead of pushed-around, little, doesn't-matter daughter-in-law. But obviously we were all so scared that we could only hit each other.

Maybe this is the time to make my apology, to make an apology for the things cancer makes us say. Everyone who knew John was so fierce about his or her desire that he live, and because trying to slap John out of his wasting was useless, we slapped each other with hurtful words. Cruelly, even though none of us was the cancer patient, we might as well have been. No tubes and IVs going through us draining tumor fluid from us or injecting chemicals into us, but instead, invisible tubes, filled with the fear that we were going to lose John, ran through us along with IVs of powerlessness that bred hate and anger toward any who might disturb our edgy balance.

There I was feeling the baby kick, as the minutes slogged by. Last week I'd written John a letter and had left it on his night table for him to read after I'd gone.

Dearest John,

Through these tough days, as we wait to hear what's going on, I can't tell you what a comfort it is to me whenever your baby gives a kick. There's quite a bit of activity tonight, and you'll think I'm nuts, but I pat my stomach and talk to it, saying that Daddy's going to be okay! I think of you all through the day—I just wish I could have some of these tests for you. I know today was a real trial to you and learning nothing as a result of these tests is happy in one way but so frustrating. I guess this is going to call on supreme patience from both of us, but of course especially from you. I know you're strong enough to accept that and will do it with the intelligent good grace you do everything. The calls sure do come in. So many people love you so much. As I told you, I had a good talk with Martha Rooney [a close friend of ours] tonight and later on David called. Just everybody is thinking of you. Be strong, my dearest one. We just have to have faith in Dr. Lisio and hope he figures this one out soon. You can imagine how I miss you. And oh how I love you!

Nancy

I looked at my watch. An hour had gone by. I went back to the needlepoint. A few minutes later the door opened. Dr. Wiedel introduced himself; was I Nancy? Yes. He was all clean and back into his pressed white coat, shirt and tie, and this was a conversation I would never forget.

He sat down on the edge of John's bed, facing me in my chair. I leaned forward and made the footrest go back into the base of the chair. He said, "I was so sorry I missed you last night. John said you'd just left. I'd wanted to have a chance to talk to you and explain what we were going to be doing today while I explained it to John. He certainly is devoted to you. He told me all about you, which made me even more regretful that I'd missed meeting you yesterday."

I smiled, nodded my head, still didn't say anything. Something was coming, I could feel it. I closed my eyes for a second and thought I must be in a movie. My heart was beating fast; I licked my dry lips.

"John," he said, "does have a tumor."

I grabbed for the notepad on John's night table and a pencil; I wanted to write everything down.

"We're pretty sure it's mesothelioma."

My notes said: "Mesothelioma?"

"But, we'll know for sure when the pathologist's report

is in. I only see about one a year of these, and I've never seen one in a thirty-three-year-old."

Oh, God. I breathed in and out as slowly as I could as I wrote all this down.

"It is malignant."

There it was, it was true, oh, God.

"We took out eight"—8, I write, 8—"quarts of fluid from the tumor. It will come back, though—the tumor will continue to produce fluid. There are two catheters in John now to help drain more off. I didn't get"—or did my notes say "take out"?—"any of the tumor."

I asked.

"Yes, that's right, I couldn't take it out. It's in the omentum—that's the lining of the abdomen. If it is mesothelioma, and we'll know by tomorrow, we'll start calling medical centers all around the country. Chemotherapy or radiotherapy may not even work. But as I said, we'll call medical centers all around the country to ask if any of them have had any success in treating this kind of tumor. We will do everything we can to save him."

I looked up at him. I tried to smile and he tried to return a hopeful smile back to me, but both of our eyebrows were pressed closed together on our faces, meeting over the bridges of our noses, the strain of holding ourselves in was showing on our contracted faces.

"How long?" I asked. "How long?" Jesus, just like they do in the fucking movies.

And I was not prepared for the answer. He'll say five years, a year, something, I thought—but he answered, "Very short, Nancy, very short."

With that I cupped my hand over my mouth and slowly breathed in a breath that stabbed me. I looked at him with terror. I took another deep breath. My face was starting to tremble of its own accord and I couldn't stop it. I quickly regained control; I had to ask more questions, I had to be sure I had heard that correctly.

"John told me you were a very strong young lady." I started to cry now. "And you are," he said. I held my head up, my chin jutted forward, I, who had just been hit in the gut, was determined to hold on, I had to, I know now, for John. I looked like a pinched-in, frightened little girl but also a regal, composed woman, a grown-up, and I stayed that way for the next eleven weeks.

I now began to understand as we continued to talk that Columbia-Presbyterian had never been able to treat mesothelioma successfully. He mentioned asbestos. If, he said, if it is mesothelioma, it is caused by asbestos. Asbestos? When had John ever been around asbestos?

Dr. Wiedel gripped my shoulder as he rose off the edge of the bed and patted me. "You're a wonderful woman. John is lucky."

The door closed silently behind him. I looked around the room. Oh, yes, I remembered, yes, he said John was now in the recovery room and would be down in a while. I looked at the clock. Not even an hour and a half had gone by since he went up there. Oh, that other thing, yes—"We sewed him back up." Very short, very short, what did it mean? Very short. And like a dummy, after he told me that, I asked again if the tumor was malignant. Yes, he said as he nodded his head.

I can't remember now what I did. I may have called my mother, I may not have. Dr. Wiedel was on his way to call John's parents. I stood in that room and looked out the window between the other medical buildings to the Hudson River, *goddam windows are still never washed in this place.* I looked at the George Washington Bridge, John's favorite bridge—he was a bridge person, and that was his favorite. I went into the bathroom and washed my face with one of the washcloths he'd used that morning. It was still damp.

And went back and stared out that window. I patted my stomach and said to myself, "I put my right hand in God's and John's hand in God's other hand and know that everything will be all right. That God will protect all of us, Daddy, Mommy and Baby."

The door opened behind me. I turned around and saw John being wheeled in. I helped the orderlies open the door farther and helped get him back into his bed off the stretcher. He looked stunned, as if hit on the head, and yet he smiled at me. He was groggy, and I was stupid; I should have realized, remembered from my own times under anesthesia how unreal the world is for a long time afterward, but I had a feeling I had to take control and tell him we had a lot to talk about.

John's face turned up to me, and he smiled, and he said, "About what, Little One?"

I practically gagged. The doctor had said John had been told exactly what I'd been told. I realized immediately that nothing could be expected in logical sequence anymore. There were no rules. And if he didn't want to talk about "it," I wouldn't make him. I kissed his forehead.

"I'm so sleepy, Nini."

"Sure, Bunky, it'll take some time for the anesthesia to wear off. How're you feeling?"

"Okay, Nini, okay."

"Good. Listen, you close your eyes and rest. I'll be sitting right here. Is there anything I can get you? Okay, fine, you rest. Yes, I'm right here."

A few minutes later Dr. Lisio came in and motioned for me to come out into the hallway with him. We walked toward the two public phone booths, away from the other rooms. He put his arm around my shoulder and then began. He went over the surgery, the results, the asbestos connection, yes, he was sure it was mesothelioma. He gripped my shoulder tighter and said, "Nancy, as Dr.

Wiedel told you, chemotherapy may not work. The best we might be able to do is to try to keep him comfortable by draining off the fluid the tumor produces." I looked up at his kind face, his glasses covering his eyes, his soft, low voice hesitating. "Our goal, Nancy, is to keep him alive to see the baby, to keep him alive long enough to see the baby."

That is what "very short" means, *that, that,* that he may not live long enough to see the *baby*? It's only until January—that's three months away. I didn't say anything, I was rocking back and forth on my feet.

Lisio took my hands in his. "One thing, Nancy, one thing you've got to remember, you must remember"—and he pulled me closer to him, our hands locked, me gripping him so tightly, crushing his fingers, his voice becoming louder, more insistent—"you've got to remember, Nancy, that *your life is going to be all right. You're going to make it. You're going to be all right.* Your life is going to be all right, all right." His voice was softer.

He was right, he was right to have said that, and I'll always be grateful to him for that. I did think my life was over, he told me it wasn't going to be, that I would survive this. Nobody will understand this, but I needed to be told that. I shook my head though, no, I shook, my life was over if it was a life without John. He pulled my head up and looked into my eyes. He shook his head back and forth and mouthed the word "No."

No, he was telling me again with his eyes and with the strong grip of his fingers around mine, no, your life isn't over, you will have a future, a good future, you must believe this. At that point I dropped my hands from his grip and put my arms around him and cried on his chest, rocking back and forth. I was getting the front of his white coat wet, I was sobbing silently, and he was holding me.

"Never," he said, "never would I have thought it would

be John Rossi. If I could see the future and were retiring from my practice tomorrow, twenty-five, thirty years from now, I would be certain that I would be giving John the name of another doctor to look after him. Of all my patients, Nancy, of all my patients, he is the one I would have placed money on to survive me and my practice by years and years."

I was buckling into his chest, my stomach, my pregnant stomach was heaving. I put my hand on it, the baby, the baby. I started to wipe my eyes with my hands, to get the tears off, I sniffled, I needed a Kleenex, he got me one. I breathed in. I was coming out of it.

"I don't know what to tell you, Nancy. I'm not even sure we should use a 'go for broke' treatment. I don't know. My own feeling is maybe to make John as comfortable as we can, drain the tumor when it's necessary."

I looked up at him. Was there no hope in his eyes? No, none. It was over. It was all over.

I went back to the room and peeked in. John was sleeping. I got my handbag and walked back to the phone booths and sat down and first called his boss, Bill Rubinstein, at work. It was afternoon now. Bill wanted to know immediately, and I called to tell him. No, no answer, the day had gone by faster than I thought, no one was answering at Kelley Drye. I called my mother. I then called Croton and got Aunt Helen and told her that their goal was to keep John alive long enough to see the baby. Esther and Vincent came on the phone. The guardrails were down between us. We cried.

I went back to the room. John was awake. Groggy still, he was being given a shot of painkiller for the incision. The bandage covered his chest. We talked quietly. About nothing, about everything. Was he feeling better? Yes. Would he like anything? Yes, a sip of water. Water was forbidden. I asked the nurse if he could have a chip of ice; I remembered that after my operations I was allowed that or even to suck on a wet washcloth. Yes, she said, the ice chip would be okay. She told John to let it melt on his tongue slowly. The worry was that they didn't want him to throw up and rip that incision open during those first hours. Yes, tomorrow he'd probably be allowed some broth. Then the next day some soft food.

I patted John's forehead and smoothed his hair back from it. Very softly. He dozed off again, and I went back to the telephones. My mother was at the hospital now. She had brought the car up and would wait in the lounge until I wanted to go home.

I called Bill at home. He answered the phone. I told him, and as I told him he started to cry and called "Sheryl, come here," to his wife, and soon they were both crying on the phone, and it may have been then or it may have been the next night, but I said to Bill that I didn't know if the firm was planning on making John a partner or not, but, and here Bill started to sob, they both did, but I asked, if it's okay, it would mean so much, you see, would they please make John a partner, it would mean so much to him, it would give him something to live for even though he wouldn't live, but I said don't do it out of pity, do it only if you were going to do it anyway. Sheryl said of course they were going to make him a partner, didn't John *know* that? No, I answered, he didn't. We hung up.

I called information and got the phone number of John's senior boss, Jack Costello, the senior partner in the tax department. Mrs. Costello answered the phone and I said hello, that John had been operated on, and could I talk to Mr. Costello. And I told him, "Their goal is to keep him alive to see the baby in January." How many times would I say that sentence in the next twenty-four hours? His voice caught in his throat, this man who seemed to terrorize and frighten so many of the associates at the firm, and he, as I kept talking, was crying, too, saying, oh, no, not John, oh, no, oh, the baby, oh, no, and then deep, deep sobs. I wanted to tell you myself, I told him. Yes, I just spoke to Bill. And to Mr. Costello, too, I begged, as I cried, I asked him please to make John a partner.

It was a dark, dark night out by now. I walked down to the end of the hall to the lounge area where my mother sat. I told her I was ready to go home, that John was sleeping, was probably asleep for the night, and we took the elevator down and I put on my raincoat and we walked up to the garage a block and a half away and I waited downstairs while Mom went a floor or two above and got the car. We didn't say anything. I assumed she'd already called my father and brother with this awful news, but I didn't even ask. I don't remember even crying. I just sat in that car as she drove me home, left me off at the door and went around to the garage to drop the car off and tell José, the garage attendant, when we'd need it the next morning. She must have told José, dear José, what had happened. José, who always had the car ready for John at seven on a Saturday or Sunday morning so that he could go pick up David Clark and drive out to Bogota, New Jersey, to play tennis at the indoor courts there. José, Mom told me, was stunned.

I returned to the apartment, and she followed soon after. I made no sense, I felt I had to call everyone I knew, personally. From dear Patsy whom I worked with at Nightingale and all John's and my Bayberries friends all the way down. And I began each call by saying that I wanted to tell them myself, that they should not hear it from someone else.

After the five or six calls were made I told Mom I was going to bed. As I was lying there, trying to think of what could be worse, I realized that with illness, at least, one has time to adjust to the fact that one is going to lose the owner of "his books, his suits, his running shorts, his bookcase," the person who chose the magical dark-blue wallpaper in the bedroom. That it wasn't like a car accident or a plane crash. Well, these goodbyes came all at once for me in the beginning and then they were over with until the day he died.

That night, later on, when I couldn't sleep and I knew my mother was asleep in the other bedroom, the baby's room, I got up out of bed and said goodbye to everything he'd ever owned, touched, loved. I wove, staggered really in a kind of cloudy, soft-touch haze, around the apartment, delicately alighting my fingers on one object, then another. His poetry books, his bathrobe, his chair, his box of Wheaties in the kitchen cupboard, talking to myself and naming each object the whole time and asking the air over and over again, "Is this awful thing happening to him?" Asking it out loud in complete bewilderment. No, it can't be, I thought. And only hours later, even before the dawn of the next day, I would start on the road of hopes and well-convinced denial, but that night I knew that, yes, it was so. My husband was going to die, and I was never going to see him again, and for that instant I looked that fact in the face and knew it.

I began to cry. I had no one. I tiptoed into my mother's room, saw she was sleeping. It must have been only a few hours before dawn, and I woke her up. As if I were still the frightened little girl who used to crawl into her and my father's and also sometimes into my brother's bed, I got under the covers of the sofa bed she was sleeping on and started to cry, my big stomach heaving, the baby quiet though. She woke up and put her arms around me, and I said, "Mom, oh, Mommy, Mom, my heart is breaking." And it's true, it was. I never felt such an accurate description of a real physical sensation. And I kept repeating through my tears that my heart was breaking. "It's like somebody has picked it up and smashed it against the wall," I said.

I stayed there with her, her holding me and crying with me and saying, "Oh, it's so awful, it's so awful, how could this happen to that dear boy, that dear man?" And then I started to quiet down as she rubbed my back, as if I were her little girl again who'd maybe come in crying from skinning her knee roller-skating in the driveway, and finally later I told her I was okay, that I was going to try to get some sleep. I walked back to the dining room and looked out the windows onto Madison Avenue, and the world seemed unreal, the taxis still going by at four in the morning were unreal, the hardware store across the street. Do people really get up and go about their errands every day? I wondered. How can they when death is in a hospital only eighty blocks away? How can they?

I went back to my bed, and then, even without a night's sleep, a peacefulness and sureness that John would survive, fight it, live for me and his child-to-be filled me in the morning as my room grew lighter. It was to keep my mind from falling apart, to keep my husband's own will to live fierce and strong; it was denying the inevitable, the beginning of absolute trust in physicians and in miracles and in God, who certainly could not let this beautiful young man die. I became a beggar at anybody's altar in the weeks ahead. Even the weather became a symbol: a bright clear day meant John would live. John McEnroe winning the Davis Cup meant John would live, a nonstop ride in the elevator up to the floor where John's room was meant that John would live, finding a penny later on the floor of the phone booth on his floor at Mt. Sinai Hospital, where he was to be transferred, meant he was going to live, wishing on stars at night meant he would live, calling the Fifth Avenue Presbyterian Church's Dial-A-Prayer and listening to Dr. Kirkland meant he would live, having a relaxed five-minute conversation with one of his doctors meant he would live, feeling the baby kick meant he would live. Desperate, grasping for any comfort. Except for one, which even back then brought a smile and a laugh of disbelief to me and John. We were given a vial of Lourdes water. It was from a very well-meaning and wonderful friend, but we didn't know what to do with it, especially me. John at least knew what it was. Another friend offered to "deep-six" it rapidly, as he put it, and we gratefully accepted and gave it to him. We could still laugh.

The eleven weeks of John's cancer were life. It was a normal life to us. A friend gave me Elisabeth Kübler-Ross's book on dying after John was operated on. There is some truth in the stages of one's reactions, his and mine: shock, anger, acceptance, but hell, anyone could have figured that out. But the talking about dying, it just doesn't happen, at least between a young husband and wife. It was not the movies, but was just our day-to-day life continuing under different circumstances. I hated it when someone referred then or even refers now to John's eleven weeks of illness as the time he was dying. He was not; he was living, and then one morning he died. And the whole time of his illness was, again, normal life to us. The IVs, the paracentesis of quarts and quarts of fluid from the tumor, the various chemotherapies, the loss of hair, the physical wasting—it was all normal life to us, because we had no choice, because we had to take the risk that one of the treatments would let him live longer, and because we knew that back there somewhere in our minds was our home. Being home together again was a goal we both dreamed of, and even in our most faithless moments of anguish, we were convinced of its certainty and reality, but our new life had equal meaning. As I kept trying to explain to people then, "It's just different."

SATURDAY, SEPTEMBER 30, 1978

Dear Bunky,

Here are lots of books for you—let me know when you want a new supply.

Don't think, my dearest, that I don't realize what a heavy dose of shit you've been handed, and so unexpectedly. But I know that after the shock has worn off, you're going to "look on the bright side" again. So many people have told me that a positive, fighting attitude has caused superior health to return to people who have cancer, and since you have more guts and the happiest attitude of anyone I know, I know you're going to pull this one out of the hat. Think about the future in a happy way, but when the going is tough, just think about each day as it comes. You never have been a worrier and you're not going to start now.

What can I say about the partnership? I am so proud of you, I'm strutting and dancing around. (I do not, however, as Leo [our cat] reminds me, dance as well as you!) Oh— there's something that Bill and Sheryl told me: they said you do the best work of anybody in the firm. How about that?! Needless to say, that's no surprise to me.

Oh—too—I have to tell you, I got the nicest note from Mrs. Conway! [Wife of one of the partners] Can you imagine? Patsy too gives her happiest hello and regards to you.

I hope you don't go back to pajamas too soon—you're as sexy as hell in that short hospital gown. Sure hope the baby gets your great legs and not my short, fat stumps! Meanwhile, I am right with you every moment. And remember that wonderful things like partnerships, babies, the house in Bridgehampton, etc., are going to keep happening to us again and again.

Love,

That's what I mean by normal life.

CHAPTER FIVE

B y the day after the operation, the pathologists in the lab confirmed the diagnosis of mesothelioma, and by the end of the day Dr. Lisio told me that John had remembered when he had been exposed to asbestos, that it had occurred during a summer job he'd had when he was twenty: for two weeks he had handled asbestos sheets, counting them and lifting them off and onto trucks into and out of the warehouse. Dr. Lisio said that John was pretty upset about it and that he thought it wiser that I not bring up the subject of asbestos but let John bring it up himself. Down the hall I could see my mother sitting next to John's father in the tenth-floor lounge. The late-afternoon sun made bright rectangles of light on the gray-and-black linoleum floor and across my father-in-law's suit. He was holding his head in his hands, shaking his head back and forth, and I could see my mother was talking to him.

I went back into John's room to find a cheerful and less groggy John, and he was looking forward to the broth that he would be allowed to eat for supper that night. Later on, my mother told me that John's father, when he heard John recall the time and nature of his exposure to asbestos, kept repeating over and over, "I can't tell his mother." He felt responsible because he had been the one who had encouraged John to take these summer jobs, jobs at companies that were clients of his law firm. And my mother was trying to tell him that he must not blame himself, that how could he or anyone have known then how dangerous asbestos was.

The next day Dr. Wiedel returned to tell us that he had located three doctors in the country who had had any success in treating mesothelioma and one of them was at Mt. Sinai Hospital in New York City. We both asked about Sloan-Kettering, knowing its reputation, but Dr. Wiedel shook his head and said that experts there felt too that John's best chances were with the doctor at Mt. Sinai, Philippe Chahinian. We were told Dr. Chahinian was from France and had worked with that country's leading oncologist, Dr. Lucien Israel. It was agreed that Dr. Chahinian would come to Harkness to meet John and discuss his treatment. Out of eight mesothelioma patients, he had written in a recent paper, two had had complete remissions. I held John's hand as we listened—this would be the escape, he would live after all.

Such good news came the day members of Kelley Drye's trust and estates department arrived with a will for John to sign and for them to witness. He'd never had a will. Sometime after we were married I'd asked him if he thought it might be wise for us both to make out wills. "Oh, no, Nini, I don't see any reason for it, at least not until we have children." Really? I'd answered. I was surprised.

How could a lawyer not have a will? But as the years passed, I stopped bringing it up; by then I'd learned that John was so frightened of dying that he was too scared to make out his own will, that he'd make one only if he were forced to, as he was that day. Now with the news about Dr. Chahinian, we smiled, thinking that maybe the will hadn't been necessary after all. And with the exciting games between the Yankees and the Red Sox for the American League Eastern Division title and John's rapid recovery from the surgery, everything was going to be, we were sure, all right.

Every day there were visitors for John, his family, my mother, me, friends from the law firm. And John learned how tiring it can be to be a host when all one wants to do is sleep or read quietly. The exhaustion of making conversation, of chatting, reacting to our comments—"You look *won*derful today, John. How do you feel?" Comments meant to keep our own spirits up as well as his, but exhausting to listen to and to answer. John would prove his improving strength by walking down the hall to the lounge and back, by taking a shower and shaving every day, by calling the firm and telling them not to forget him, that he was still capable of answering questions that might come up in his work, which temporarily had been assigned to another associate, by refusing to take all the Percodan painkiller tablets that were prescribed to him each day.

He and I both remembered a man who worked in the tax department of Chrysler out in Detroit, whom John had worked with and liked very much, and who a couple of years before had had a heart attack, followed by open-heart surgery. He had told John that it was as if the guys in the office had thought he was already dead, the way they treated him, not recounting office news, just assuming that he'd ceased to exist, that he'd never come back to work. These things, he'd said to John, were worse than the actual heart attack and surgery. It was only recently, after he'd been back at work for just about two years, that his colleagues didn't give him the impression that he might not be able to handle a difficult workload, that he might croak any minute.

Some of the visitors John had would glance at him when they arrived, turn their faces downward, and then, after chatting and talking, when they were about to leave, glance over at me, a look full of pity. Impossible to stand up and tell them, "We don't want to be pitied! Please try to treat us the way you always have!" But of course neither John nor I could open our mouths to say it. It seemed the visitors were more in control than we were, that we both still had to react the same way to talk about the weather but that they couldn't react the same way to us, and we were going to have to adjust to that. John and I talked about this, and John once laughed and said, "I was about to whisper to you, Nini, to get them out of here!" I know that to see a grown man in a hospital gown, when one is used to seeing him dressed for work or tennis, is shocking. The hospital gown, instead of conferring almost feminine fragility, as it does to a woman, gives a childlike look to a man. And maybe that's what threw the visitors, maybe not so much how he looked, but that he was in a hospital gown.

On one of these bright early-October days two of John's cousins came in to see him, and they offered to take him outside for a walk. John got so excited, he appreciated it so much. He got permission from the nurse, and she got a wheelchair for him to ride down the elevator in. He sat down in it in his bathroom and practically yelled, "Yippee, let's go!" as he put his feet into his slippers. His mother insisted that he put a blanket over his lap, and John refused—after all, David and Peter were in shirts and jeans, it couldn't be that cold out. But she continued to insist, and John realized it would be easier to agree. He looked over at me as David wheeled him out, a furious glare, and I closed my eyes and then opened my eyes and imperceptibly nodded my head. He knew what I meant, and I knew what he meant. He was angry that his adult judgment was in question, and I knew it, and I knew he'd given in for the sake of peace, that he loved his mother and didn't want to argue with her. But what it took out of him to do that!

He and his cousins were outside for a fairly long time. John even walked around the pathways in the small garden that surrounds the chapel. His father and his Uncle Jack joined them in the garden while his aunt and mother and I talked upstairs in his room. John was beaming when he returned, and I noticed that his bathrobe was loosened and that the blanket was thrown over the arm of the wheelchair. Good for you, I thought.

The Yankees–Red Sox playoff game for the American League Eastern Division title was one of the most exciting baseball games John or I had ever seen. And although I was sad the Red Sox lost, I knew that at least John would have the Series to watch against Kansas City for the league pennant. On Tuesday, October 3, we sat in his room and watched the Yankees smash Kansas City 7–1. Then on Wednesday we saw them lose 10–4—John, pounding his fist on the arm of the reclining chair in the corner and slapping his hand to his forehead, rolling his eyes up to the ceiling and asking, "Why, goddam it, do those guys swing at every first pitch?!"

October 5 was a travel day, and that was the day that Dr. Chahinian from Mt. Sinai came up to talk to John and me and to explain his treatment. Yes, John, there will be toxic side effects, yes, your hair will fall out. John asked what the doctor thought about other options, and Chahinian replied, "John, you don't have any other options."

John nodded his head and said, "Okay, how soon can you get me admitted, Doctor?"
Saturday, the 7th.

It was time now to write my friend Lizzie, a girl I'd grown up with and gone to school with, who now was living in London with her husband. The last letter I had written her was in August when they had just moved there from New York, her husband having been transferred to London by Chase Manhattan for two or three years. *She won't believe this. She just won't believe this.* I wrote in part:

OCTOBER 12, 1978

Dear Lizzie,

  . . . As it has turned out, there are three men in the United States who have been treating this kind of cancer, and one is at Mt. Sinai. He came up and saw John and me at Presbyterian to explain the chemotherapy he uses, the side effects, etc., and John has since been moved to Mt. Sinai and is now one of this man's 30 patients. His rate of "success" is really remarkable; and he was able to give us the following figures: 25% of his cases have had complete remissions; 35% have resulted in the tumor being stabilized; the remaining 40% were not helped, but he then has gone on to other drugs, and is also researching immunotherapy. We'll know after John's third treatment what group he fits in. His treatments last 5 days every three weeks in the hospital. Two drugs are fed into him intravenously 24 hours a day. One drug is experimental, but as the nurse told us, it's not considered very experimental on his floor, as it's been around two years, because most of the other patients on his floor are on drugs that have only been previously used on animals.

John's unit in the hospital looks like something out of
Star Trek! There are only 19 beds, and the patients and
staff are the most cheerful people in the world. Many of the
patients are as young as John. The worst thing for me has
been his incredible loss of weight. He has gone from about
175 lbs. in August to now about 120 lbs. It is awful. His
stomach is terribly distended from the fluid the tumor produces, and, of course, he is still recovering from the surgery. The incision is about 10 inches long up and down his
stomach. Occasionally he gets the fluid tapped out of him,
but they can't do it very often. The result is terrible pains in
his back from the pressure of the fluid on his spinal column.

It's all happened so fast that he hasn't adjusted to all of it
(not that I have!), but I'm hoping that his normal good spirits plus some fight will return to him. Hopefully, he will be
coming home this weekend, and that should cheer him up.
Then he'll be an out-patient for the three weeks in between
treatments when he will have his blood count taken often,
etc. Also during these first three weeks his hair will fall out.

As you can imagine, it's been a nightmare. The thought
of being a widow and bringing up a child by myself is still
very unreal to me. At least, though, his baby will give me
something to live for, otherwise I'd probably be in the East
River. I naively thought that our years of trying to have
children were some of the worst times I'd lived through—
they seem positively gay in retrospect. Nothing can replace
a husband. . . .

I wish you were here to talk to. I'm actually a lot more
hopeful than I sound in this letter. Some days are good and
some bad—this one not a particularly good one as John was
in an awful lot of pain when I saw him. But I've learned
that another day with him no matter what it holds is a real
gift. One note of humor that you'll appreciate, though: you
know how fond I am of John's parents, and his father's been
pretty good, if glum, but his mother has been more difficult.

Jesus, dealing with them on top of the rest of it, when they're determined to see everything in the gloomiest possible way, has been a real trial. I had to insist that they not be there with me during his operation and that I wanted to get the results of the operation first. For a while there they were trying to kick me out of the picture and have the doctors deal only with them. Some strong words have come from me that I never thought I'd have the courage to say, and you know what, they are now behaving! It's made me feel I've really accomplished something.

All my love to you and Woody. Take care of yourself, and hopefully in the next six weeks I'll be able to write with some good news.

Nancy

How to explain Lizzie and myself? Both of us short and always in the first row of any class photograph. Both of us always trying to lose that extra five pounds, which on our small frames looked more like ten. In that regard those extra pounds have turned into ten for me, and Lizzie lost those five pounds and more.

We went to school together, and I remember that on my first day in seventh grade at my first gym class, Lizzie and I made a pact. The gym teacher was about to start us off playing dodge ball, and not even knowing each other yet—I was new; she'd been there since kindergarten—we promised that we'd never hit each other with a dodge ball. And we never did.

We liked each other all right during those school years, but both of us had closer friendships with others in our class. There were only fifteen girls in our whole grade, and friendships shifted very slowly. It just was too obvious if one wanted to end or begin a friendship. So we pretty much stayed within very small groups, though the class as a whole actually loved one another very much. I don't remember anybody being deliberately cruel to another, maybe ignoring but not cruel.

Lizzie was much more of a scholar than I was. I worked just as hard, but the result of my work didn't have that solid ring of authority that hers had. I posed a lot of questions in my papers, suppositions, with not too many facts to back them up, and never really answered too many of the questions I'd raised, but I loved taking one side and then another and going back and forth—in other words, talking. Lizzie's papers could have been read at a General Assembly meeting of the UN and made sense, whereas mine were more suited to an off-Broadway stage. Oddly, we pretty much got the same grades in school, especially in math, in which we were both lousy. She won out in history, and I did a little better in English, and we both stayed pretty equal in French, Latin and science.

I think our classmates liked us both a lot. Both of us were able to be friendly with each small group in our class, which probably was the reason we both held a number of offices during the years. I remember Lizzie as being fairly relaxed and sure and controlled about her work and whatever else occupied her time at school. I was more fidgety, doubtful and passionate about my work and my outside interests. I remember that during review week before our final exams one high school year, I, instead of reviewing anything, read the plays of George S. Kaufman and Moss Hart and wound up cramming hours before exams. My interests then would alight on something, some subject, some art, some person, and I would do nothing else until I had learned and read all I could about it. We had many characteristics in common, but probably the major one was a sense of organization, which probably also helped us win all those elections. Both of us could run a meeting, dole out jobs and errands to people on a committee working on a project, and keep an accurate sheet of what had been done and what hadn't.

Our families were different. Hers was a large family, with older sisters and a brother who had children by the time she was in high school, and her parents, and Lizzie had a twin sister as well. I had one older brother, also married, and my parents were divorced. Lizzie's family had trust funds, mine didn't. I can remember spending a few weekends with Lizzie's family, which to me was like walking into a Walt Disney movie. Everybody was lovely, intelligent, genuinely interested in the events of the day of each member of the family, and they were also very controlled and beautifully behaved. Things moved at a very nice, calm pace in that household. Mine was very different. Before my parents separated, their nights were filled with drinking and yelling. During the day my mother rarely went outside, or barely even got out of bed. I did most of the shopping for food and learned early to cook for myself. My mother went up to the roof of our building a couple of times, weavingly drunk, yelling at my father with one leg over the railing of the twenty-first floor and saying she was going to jump. My brother was away at college then, so he missed the last years of our parents' marriage. But once my mother and I moved to another apartment, and she and my father were divorced, things improved enough so that I could have friends over, and my mother even got a job and returned more actively to life. By my first year in college, my father had stopped drinking completely. And today, although divorced, my parents get along extraordinarily well. Neither remarried, and their common bond now is their grandchildren.

The idea of the two families ever getting together then was out of the question. Actually it was that way with the families of every member of my class. We were an odd assortment of girls. Lizzie's family and one other were the most normal of the fifteen families. The girls mixed around a bit, but except for picking up their daughters at birthday parties and later dances, the parents had little to do with each other.

Very quickly I'll say that I was the first vice-president of the school not to be elected president the following year. Lizzie ran against me, there was a tie, a revote, and she won. At the time it seemed like the end of my life. It was because I was liked and respected and popular at school, that I had been able to cope with the mess at home, with living with my mother. I was the most graceless loser imaginable: I cried during a math class with Lizzie sitting a few seats away, and I recall I eventually ran out of the school and met my brother down at the Plaza.

I'm surprised Lizzie and I ever spoke to each other again, but we had developed another common bond aside from dodge ball in our senior year. We watched in horror as our classmates went to Central Park to smoke marijuana. This was 1966–67. One of our friends had a boyfriend who was a student at Columbia University. Let me mention that boys were nonexistent in our lives; girls in the classes above us and below us managed to date and even have steady boyfriends, whereas my classmates usually went to dances with someone's cousin dragged in from New Jersey who was five foot three at the most and smelled. There were a few collegiate boys who followed our class around, but Lizzie and I, along with at least eight others in our class, thought they were drips. We were a very picky bunch, except for a set of twins who went out with the local pizza-delivery boys, but all of us would have leaped to go out with someone at Columbia, so you can imagine the collective pride we all felt that one of our number had accomplished just that, and he wasn't just a one-time date, he was a boyfriend and our friend had even slept with him! My God, we were proud of her!

Sure, we were a little jealous, too, but mostly we all were so pleased that at least one of us had made it and made it with someone we all agreed was the epitome of what we felt a man should be. I think a few others in the class had slept with someone, but I can guarantee for the most part that their partners were people they never wanted to see again and people they never would have shown off to the rest of us, or else, and this was probably more likely, they slept with boys who never called *them* back afterward. Anyway, this was something Lizzie and I never had to worry about, as nobody had even asked us, and the ones who might possibly have done so were so completely out of the question that it was a closed subject for us. Hell, I'm assuming this—maybe Lizzie had a secret hot romance—but I'm sure our virginity didn't leave us until pretty much the same time in college.

You should now have the picture that dating a Columbia boy was equal to having Zeus call one of us up to Olympus for a short roll. It was that far away and that unlikely. Our friend learned a lot at Columbia, in the dorms of her boyfriend's friends and in their apartments, and she brought back stories of people smoking marijuana. We didn't even know how to say it. We were all fascinated, but only a few of us tried any when we were brought some joints.

This was long before the concerts in the park with a permanent purple haze of grass in the air; this was when people were getting arrested, busted, jailed. I am sure Lizzie and I probably would have tried grass then if we weren't so scared about its illegality. Neither of us wanted to get arrested. I have a theory that there are two groups of people: those who got caught at everything at school—note-passing, yawning during assembly, cutting gym—and those who got away with anything they tried. Lizzie and I were charter members of the first group, which is probably the third reason why we were so easily electable. Lizzie and I just knew in the deepest parts of our hearts that all we'd have to do was reach for a joint, or even just be there along with the others, and the police would tap us, not the others, on the shoulder and take us away. No question.

Neither of us, as I recall, got into our "first-choice" college that senior year, and neither of us stayed at the college we wound up going to for more than a couple of years. She was in Baltimore, and I was in Boulder at two very different kinds of schools, but we both went through some very hard times at the same time. Not many in the class are even married now, but Lizzie was the second in the class to get married, and her life settled into a comfortable life with a wonderful man. I married about three years later, and we had one more thing in common, really the most important thing two women could have in common: a sparkling, shining, happy, rewarding, successful marriage. This put us somewhat apart from our class. Then another classmate got married, and the three of us had something else in common that was crucial to all of us: none of us could have children, it seemed.

For a while in 1977 I can remember the three of us trading information. Did Clomid work for you? Have you had a laparoscopy to scrape your tubes? Does your temperature chart show that you ovulate? The three of us could have written a book on infertility, and we probably should have.

Time and Dr. Uscher finally found the cure of a hormone for me; Lizzie, the one who'd endured the most pain with hormone treatments, the one who had gone through the most years without conceiving, was resigned to the fact that nothing would work for her, but, a miracle, in August 1981; she gave birth to a baby girl.

John's transfer to Mt. Sinai made one aspect of life easier: I would no longer have to travel up to 168th Street, my mother driving the car every day, parking it in the garage there, then driving back downtown. Mt. Sinai was only ten blocks away, and I could walk. As enthusiastic as I sounded to Lizzie in my letter about John's ward, the 6 North Department of Neoplastic Diseases, I think it scared John the day my mother and I drove him there. John had gotten dressed in his gray flannel pants, which barely could fit around his waist—in fact, he left the top unbuttoned and loosely buckled his belt over the gap—and he wore a shirt and tie and his blue blazer. He sat up in the front seat next to my mother, who drove, and I could tell from the back that every bump and pothole in the road was going right through him. I also think he was scared. There was no turning back now. He was going to go ahead with Dr. Chahinian's treatments, he had no other choice.

Knowing him so well, I'm sure that must have bothered him, feeling he had no other choice. Being a lawyer, John always had choices, to use or not use information or evidence, to make a decision one way or another. Here had been the ultimate question: live possibly three months, having the tumor fluid tapped periodically, or risk even more for a slim chance of a life that might include a remission. If he'd been an old man, his work and family obligations behind him, a man who'd seen his grandchildren, maybe he would have decided on the first, to live as painlessly as possible and just wait out the three months for the inevitable. But here was a man with a child on the way, a young wife, a wonderful future as a partner in his law firm.

I sometimes think that maybe he made the decision in

favor of the treatments because of me, because he knew
how frightened I'd be if left alone without him. I wonder,
and this is only a guess, if even with all the future in front
of him, *he* would have preferred not taking the risk and
instead leaving with me immediately to see the Pyramids
in Egypt. He so wanted to see them and other Egyptian
antiquities, and the next three months would be his last
chance. He brought it up only once, when two months
later he was so weak that even calling off treatment then
would not have given him the strength to travel, but he
did say, "Nini, I do wish I had seen the Pyramids." How I
wish I could have given him that before he died, but I
made a vow that I would someday take our little girl or
boy to see them for him.

I remember when we got to Mt. Sinai, John sat in a chair
in the crowded waiting room until the administrative staff
behind the check-in desk called John's name. As the minutes went by, John became more and more uncomfortable.
After thirty minutes, I went back up to the desk and insisted that John be admitted immediately. I told them
again to what department he was being admitted and that
he was obviously in pain, and couldn't someone get him
to his room while I waited to fill out the necessary forms
for admission. Well, they didn't know, it was usually not
done, you know.

I was standing in front of the glass partition that separated me from the woman behind it, leaning my hands on
the counter in front of me, my pregnant stomach in front
of her eyes, and I told her to look over there, to the man in
the chair next to the window, and I told her, "That's my
husband. He's to start chemotherapy treatments with
Dr. Chahinian. We've just come down from Columbia-
Presbyterian, where he's been for the past three weeks,
and we were told that he would be admitted immediately." I was fierce and stared at her with unblinking eyes.

She turned to look at John, who was staring ahead of him just trying to bear the pain of sitting in that plastic molded chair for another minute and another minute after that. His eyes then closed—maybe it was easier that way—and the woman behind the desk turned her eyes back to me and my stomach. She said: "I'll get an aide right away to take him up in a wheelchair." She gave me the forms to fill out, John's full name, place of birth, mother's maiden name, father's name, religion, etc., etc., Blue Cross and Blue Shield numbers, his Social Security number. I knew all of this information by heart, and began to fill in the forms as fast as I could.

The man with the wheelchair appeared in another ten minutes. I had to tap John gently on the shoulder. He opened his eyes; there was a vagueness about them and what they were seeing. He got up slowly, the others in the waiting room now looking at him—this was the first wheelchair to be seen—and an old fat couple sitting on the welded-to-the-floor plastic chairs in the middle of the room said to one another in grainy, whiny voices, loud enough for me, John and everyone to hear, "Oh, how awful. He doesn't look good. He must be really sick!" John slid down into the wheelchair, his arms lowering himself slowly onto the seat, and he looked down at his shoes. Even the few children in the room stared at him, at that huge stomach, at that gaunt head. We didn't say a word. I stood right next to him as the aide began to push John out to the elevators. You bet, I thought to myself, glancing over at the couple, you bet he doesn't look good. He scares you, doesn't he? And it made me sick to think that that fat nosy woman and her husband who kept nodding his head were probably going to live a lot longer than John would get the chance to.

When we got off the elevator on the sixth floor, we turned around the corner to a pair of swinging doors with a sign in white modern block lettering on an orange background over the door: Department of Neoplastic Diseases. We passed through the doors and walked past a lounge-waiting room on the left, upholstered chairs and sofa in a soft suede-like fabric in brown and tan, their wooden arms and frames with a smooth finish, flecked-tweed carpeting on the floor, a color television anchored from the ceiling. As we walked by, there was a man watching the television, his IV bottles and monitoring machine attached to the portable pole next to him, a bathrobe over his hospital gown, his face not too pale, not too thin, no hair on his head. He looked up and nodded a greeting as we passed. The one public telephone was outside the room. A water fountain on the left as we continued down the hall to the nurses' station. A high counter in the middle of the floor, patients' charts kept in blue plastic binders behind on a bookshelf, each identified by a wide strip of masking tape marked with the patient's last name in thick black marker.

Yes, John's room was ready. We were led farther down the hall. The patients' semiprivate rooms were all on the left. Some of the doors were open, some half closed, some shut. I saw a woman sitting on her bed, in a pretty night-gown, talking on the phone, her children sitting around her, her husband, too. Looked as if they were in their fifties. Patches of wispy hair on her head; most of the hair had come out. John's room was the last one on the left, 624. There were two beds, "A" next to the door and the room's bathroom, and "B" next to the window. John had the "B" bed. There was a pleasant-looking man in the "A" bed, already hooked up to his IV. Still had all his hair.

Across the hall was a sign that indicated the Wood Foundation had donated an area of the ward. It was the leukemia treatment room. There were two or three beds in there, hard to see, all enclosed in plastic. Nurses went in with gloves on their hands; everything had to be absolutely sterile there; the enclosed plastic shelters around each bed were to keep in the filtered air and keep out the possibility of infections. Another big room next to it, must have been the only private room on the floor. A young man was in there on his bed, sitting and talking with some friends. A radio was playing the Beatles, his door was covered with get-well cards taped to it. Couldn't be any older than twenty-three. No hair. It was starting to look normal.

In John's room I unpacked his suitcase, and he quickly got out of his confining clothes and into his pajamas and looked out the window. It overlooked a small plaza with a statue below. Directly in front was the new Gustave L. Levy building, a monster of a structure rising over thirty stories at the northern end of Central Park and darkening with age, the treated steel turning brown and rusty-looking, the windows tinted. (When John and I used to take weekend walks around the park and at some point look at the view from the "castle" where the weather station is, we would watch with anger as that dark building grew taller and taller, until, when it was finished, it ruined the skyline. A big black box.) To the far right out of John's window we could see the park. It was a Saturday and we could see families playing football on the grass beyond.

The man in the next bed introduced himself, and while he and John talked, I put John's toothbrush and toothpaste, razor and shaving cream into the bathroom cabinet on the side opposite Mr. S's. A nurse came in—her name was Heidi—and she told us John might be a candidate for an experiment using marijuana (in pill form) to minimize the side effect of nausea from the chemotherapy. We smiled at each other and laughed. It was just that neither of us had ever really liked marijuana.

The last time I had had any was in 1968, but John, at parties at least, where it was commonplace, would smoke with the others, as I smiled and said no thank you, that I

must be the only person in the world who is allergic to the
stuff, but it makes me sick.

What I didn't tell them was that the last time I had some
grass it had, unknown to me, but fully known to the girl
who was smoking it with me, been laced with LSD. I spent
a night wandering around Boulder, Colorado, not knowing where I was except that I thought the only way to
safety would be to find a church, the Episcopal church. I
crossed a highway, walked on the median, then realized
where I was, in the center of a highway, and I couldn't
judge the distance of the headlights coming toward me.
Could I run across to the other side? I couldn't feel my
legs, I couldn't feel my feet land when I took a step. I just
knew I had to get to that church. I ran back across the
highway and a while later started to recognize some buildings, the engineering complex—the church wasn't far
away from that, was it? I couldn't keep on the paths and
sidewalks, I kept veering off onto the grass. At last I saw
the church, and it looked as if a light was on inside, shining through the modern stained-glass windows, but when
I got there the doors were locked. I even tried the side
doors. All locked, even had link chains locked through
their door handles. I've never felt so alone. I wouldn't go
back to my dorm, not yet. The girl with whom I'd smoked
the grass had tried locking me in her room with her, and
she started at one point to put her arms around me, and
by then I knew what was happening and told her to let me
get the hell out of there. I had crawled out her window,
which was on the basement floor of the dorm, and then
crawled up the grass ledge that would get me to the lawn
in front of the dorm, she calling after for me to please
come back. While I was sitting in her room, both of us so
spaced out from this grass, in a dorm empty on a Saturday
night, she began saying that I was starting to talk funny,
that my speech was very, very, v-e-r-y slow. No, it isn't, I

said back as fast as I could say it. Was my talking slow? Then she started telling me other things, that I was looking different, and on and on, while I was saying, no, I'm still the same, but not believing that anymore, that it was just grass after all, I was okay, and then she said, "Oh, didn't I tell you? It was soaked in acid."

Then she made the move to put her arms around me to comfort me for having slipped off the end of reality, and then, God, it couldn't be true, yup, she was going to try to kiss me. LSD and a lesbian in one night. When people would ridicule me after that for not having "some of this great stuff, man, no kidding, it is g-r-e-a-tttt," I could never believe that the "great stuff" might not also have something more than marijuana in it.

So when Heidi winked at us, thinking we surely were the with-it young couple she saw in front of her, we laughed because we realized that she expected John to say, "Wow, man, all right!" when he would probably have gotten just as excited if she had told him he'd be given kelp. She then took his medical history, told him how to call to get the tiny television that swings out on a metal arm over the bed hooked up. Because the checking-in had taken so long, and John hadn't had any lunch, he asked her if he could get something to eat. She returned telling us that she didn't think she would be able to get him anything before dinner was brought around at six, but she would try, and at least she definitely had his name on the dinner list for that night.

When she left, John poured himself some ice water. What could he have been thinking? I was thinking about Heidi's telling us that the drugs John would be given weren't really experimental—"they've been around for a couple of years. Most people on this floor are on drugs previously used only on animals." In a way it was the reassurance I needed that John was in the best possible place, that a pioneering treatment might work for him, but it also made it clear that this floor was the last outpost of hope, a cheerfully decorated and antiseptic last-chance hotel, and I bet John picked that up, too.

Only the previous week in John's room in Harkness with Bill and Sheryl we had all been drinking out of the hospital glasses from the bathroom the champagne they had brought up, and Bill had been toasting John, saying congratulations to the new partner of Kelley Drye & Warren! Yes, he'd made it. "Oh, no, John, there was never a doubt, never a doubt at all!" said Bill. "You don't have to worry, John, it's official."

The grin on John's face—he hadn't looked so happy since the summer, and after asking the doctor if he could drink the champagne, and being told sure, he had been sitting on that bed at first sipping slowly—he hadn't had any alcohol for three weeks, hadn't even wanted any, and his first taste of the champagne was guarded. But he winked and said maybe he could get the doctors to let him drink this more often. "Boy, not bad," he said. "I could get used to this." He was my old party-going, laughing husband again. I was so pleased, so proud. The partnership took over everything; no one in that room was even thinking why John was there and of his future treatments. The funny congratulations card from Sheryl was passed around. It was more like a party on the maternity floor, and it was to become in the weeks ahead one of the rare times when John was treated by everyone present as a normal human being. Oh, that partnership, how much it meant to him! I'd be able, I realized, sitting there, to give him the new briefcase when he came home.

John now was talking to his roommate in the other bed. The two of them, one already hooked up to his medication, the other one about to be, were talking like two businessmen. The other man had found out that John was a lawyer, and John had found out this guy was with a bank. The man was talking about his teenage children, he had had a visit from them that morning, and then he looked at John and told him he was lucky and went on to say that he had been divorced a couple of years and that John was lucky to have a wife, that he had someone to complain to if and when the treatments got "real bad. I'll tell you," he said, "going through something like this is no fun alone. But at least I've got my kids. They're awfully good about visiting me when I come in here for these treatments."

And he nodded his head toward me. "Your first?" he asked.

"Yes," I said.

"Yes," said John, "due in January."

"That's great. Congratulations."

John asked him how long his treatment would last; he paused and then said that if his blood count was okay, he'd be finished the day after tomorrow and would be able to leave then. Then he said he was a little drowsy and asked me to pull the curtain that was attached to the metal track on the ceiling around his bed. "Your talking won't bother me," he assured us. "I'll be asleep in a flash."

I pulled up the turquoise plastic-cushioned chair to the side of John's bed. "What do you think, Bunk? Looks like a pretty fancy place."

Dumb thing to say, for John answered abruptly, "It's okay."

God, what could he have said? We were looking at that Mt. Sinai ward with two very different pairs of eyes; mine were determined to see in the space-age machinery and polished steel the best of modern medicine; his eyes must have registered, looking around, a feeling of "It's come to this. I really do have cancer. I really will be hooked up to a machine like the guy in the next bed." How terrified he must have been. But he wouldn't allow himself to linger over or even speak out loud these thoughts when I was there.

Instead, he snapped his fingers and said, "Hey, Nini, you know what I'd like to do before you leave?"

"What, Bunk?"

"Remember that memo I got from the tax department the other day? I think it's in my suitcase. Do me a favor, let me dictate an answer to you, then you can type it up at school and I'll sign it. Would that be okay?"

"Sure, John, sure."

I was smiling because he was happy and enthusiastic about something and because he needed me, I could be of use. I opened the closet door, dug in his suitcase and passed the memo to John's outstretched hand. Reading it, he started to laugh:

MEMORANDUM TO MR. ROSSI

Re: Work Load of KD&W Tax Associates

The KD&W tax associates are all furious over your prolonged absence from the firm. Although certain advantages flow from your not being here, such as the general calm which one gains from not hearing "Baby Face" continually whistled in the halls, in most respects life at KD has become burdensome and miserable. The level of work which we have been forced to take on in your absence has increased to the point of absurdity. Our usual two-hour three-martini lunches have been cut back to an hour and a half and a beer, and afternoon tea has been eliminated. We feel that these actions constitute an unfair labor practice on the part of the firm. The only conceivable remedy is for you to pull yourself together and return to work at once.

Along with the note they'd sent a few joke presents:

hand-held puzzle games he could play in bed, an instruction book on how to do origami, paper included, and a plastic pipe to blow bubbles with the bottle of bubbles. John settled back against the pillows, thought a moment, then said, "Okay, Little One, let's see how good your shorthand is," and began talking.

I wish I had a copy of what he wrote back, something about their being able to take the responsibility for anything that might go wrong in the office during his absence, his saying that he planned to return to the office in a couple of weeks, but what I remember most was how dry my throat became as I wrote down the last sentence. He said, "I miss you all very much," softly, blinking his eyes, sharply looking out the window and clearing his throat.

I was afraid he was going to start to cry, and instead of saying something like "Boy, it's rough, isn't it?" I immediately felt I had to change the atmosphere by brightly saying, "I'll have it typed for you after the weekend. You still want me and Granny to go out to the house?" I continued, "I'd much rather stay here."

"No, you go, Little One, I want you to check the house. Look, do me a favor. There's some stuff out there I'd really like, you know, my summer bathrobe, the two new mysteries I bought in East Hampton, they're on the table next to my side of the bed. Okay?" I nodded.

"Okay, good, now give me a kiss. I'll be fine, yeah, I've got money for the TV rental guy, wallet's in the drawer, no, you go, think I'll take a little nap myself until supper comes. You've got the number on the phone, right? Yeah, call when you get there. Now be a good girl, Nini, I'll see you on Tuesday."

Oh, boy, I really didn't want to go. It was the Saturday of the long Columbus Day weekend, and my mother thought it would be good for me to get away to the house in Bridgehampton for the rest of the weekend, and John, too, thought I should go. I could be very clear about exactly what was written on those drug release forms that John had signed earlier, before the chemotherapy could start, and clear, too, when listening to the doctors, but I was losing the ability to make decisions that concerned anything outside the hospital. So if John and my mother thought I should spend a couple of days in Bridgehampton, I would go, and with John's list in my pocket I could feel I was doing it for him.

It was a mistake. Driving into the driveway, walking through the house just as we'd left it on Labor Day weekend, walking on the beach in that incessantly beautiful October sunshine, on a beach I wanted to believe John would see again but wasn't sure he would. I just wished I hadn't gone. But one thing I felt I had to do out there if I did nothing else was to have my mother take a picture of me standing on the beach, with the sand and water behind me, for John to have on his night table. I look at that photograph now. My hands look as if they are pulling an invisible string apart, trying to stretch that string until it snaps, and the smile and look in my eyes, as the wind blows over my face and blows back my hair, make me look, too, as if I am ready to snap. I remember the moment before I gave my mother the camera, I was afraid I was going to cry, but quickly I stretched that smile on my face and put a gleaming imp look into my tired, aching eyes, and the result wasn't bad.

I wrote John a note to go along with it, a "have courage" note, a pep talk that he would be strong enough to withstand the treatments, and as soon as we got back to New York on Monday afternoon I put that Polaroid photograph into a plastic dime-store stand-up frame and wrote "Monday, October 9, Bridgehampton Beach" on the border. It seemed absolutely necessary that he have a picture of me on his beach, that maybe looking at it, at the place and person he loved most, would make him strong, give him the incentive to endure the chemotherapy, that maybe, maybe we would walk on that beach together if he could just hang on and fight.

My mother asked if I would like her to deliver the photograph and my note to John right away that evening. Oh, yes, would she? It would mean so much to me to know that he had my picture next to him by his bed that night. When she left, I started to cry and began writing in my diary again. A simple entry: "I have kept it in too long," followed by the facts.

The telephone rang. It was John. My mother had just left, he said. "It's a wonderful photograph of you, Little One. I've got it right here beside me. It's just what I need. You okay?" (I was scared he could tell I'd been crying.) "I love you, too, Nini. Now sleep tight; I'll see you in the morning. And it looks like I'll be out of here by the weekend! Isn't that good news?"

The first treatment went well. Although attached by IVs to the tubes and bottles and monitoring machine, he, like the man we'd seen in the lounge, could move around the room, walk to the bathroom, sit in a chair and read. It was easier than either of us had expected, and he wasn't troubled by nausea even. We were amazed. But it wasn't until John came home that the side effects would begin.

I wanted everything to be perfect for John when he returned home from Mt. Sinai after his first chemotherapy treatment. He'd been in a hospital for a full month, first at Presbyterian and then at Mt. Sinai, and his coming home at last was the gift of my life. I must have known that the next three weeks together in our home, before his next hospital treatment, would come as close to approximating our normal married life as any we'd have in the short future we had left together. And I wanted it to be perfect for him.

John tried his very strongest, but disappointments were a part of every day. There were restrictions on John's diet. He was not allowed to have salt, because that increased the build-up of fluid, which swelled his legs and feet, or anything too rich in fat or oil. If he was looking forward to one thing on his return home, it was to eat non-hospital food. He had particular cravings for Parmesan and sharp cheddar cheese, for pizza, for corned-beef hash, for anchovies. And he couldn't have any of them. But the biggest disappointment was that even foods he'd enjoyed in the past and was still allowed to eat didn't taste the same to him: fresh tomato soup, carrot soup, Wheaties cereal. The chemotherapy had distorted the taste of just about every food. At first he was so cheerful about it and would think of other things one after another that might appeal to him. And at first in my anxiousness to please him I thought of nothing but going to the supermarket as many times a day as necessary to buy any last-minute request. We both knew he had to regain weight in order to strengthen himself for the next treatment.

I never even thought about the baby during those weeks. All of my energies went to seeing that John was comfortable and had anything he wanted. I remember requesting at one point, though, that he make a list of foods he wanted me to buy so that I could shop once a day. But so often he'd remember something he'd forgotten that he'd really like right now, "if it's okay, Nini," and I'd run down to the A&P and get it for him. It didn't matter. I adored him.

One day he complained that the traffic noise on Madison Avenue was too loud during the day and said that he thought a pair of earphones connected to our stereo would be ideal so that he could listen to WQXR in peace. We were so low on cash because of the many doctor bills we had to pay prior to receiving the medical-insurance reimbursements, even with John's father's general financial aid, that I knew I'd have to go to the 86th Street Gimbels, where we had a charge account, to buy them. John knew this was a small but certain show of love for him: I hate department stores, and I hate the crowds that bring on a thick, dusty cloud of claustrophobia around me. Only at Christmastime, with the happy spirit on everyone's face, the brisk cold weather and the secure joy in my heart that comes from knowing I've thought of perfect presents for everyone in the family, does my fear dissolve. Looking at my sick John, all my phobias became insignificant. To do anything for this man was so much more important than myself.

So I went to Gimbels and bought him the earphones. I brought them home very pleased with them and myself, but as soon as John took them out of the box, he said, "These are too big, Nini, they're too heavy." And he was right. He put them on his hair-fallen-out head, which seemed so small, so thin, and the pain was unbearable for him. "Take them back. I can't stand too much weight on my head." I hadn't thought of that and said of course I'd return them right away. But I was hurt by his brusqueness, his irritability. This wasn't my John. It was his curt sharpness that hurt.

By the time I got back to Gimbels, there were endless lines and endless confusion, as the crowds of the day had arrived. Did I want to return the earphones? Yes, for an exchange. Well, that will have to be handled through the return desk. One employee and line after another until I finally had a receipt proving the return and credit for the first set of earphones. Then back to the audio counter to look for a more lightweight set. One seemed perfect to me, and although they were much more expensive, I decided to get them for John. They were a good brand, and I was sure John would be pleased with them.

He was, when I got them home, but there was a problem: they didn't work. The woman had shown and demonstrated the floor model to me, and when I had decided that I would buy them, she had gone back to the stockroom to get a new pair in an unopened box. It hadn't occurred to me to ask her to take them out of the box so that we could make sure they worked. And, as I said, John *was* pleased, and in a much better humor, really appreciative. Such a dramatic change from earlier that morning. He was so excited that they weighed so little and didn't hurt his gaunt, thin head, but as I plugged them into the stereo, one side produced only the faintest sound, no matter how high I turned the volume, and the other earphone didn't work at all. Jesus Christ, I thought to myself, I've got to go back and exchange *this* pair.

But before I went back to Gimbels, I fixed lunch for John. He particularly liked fresh grapefruit halves with honey on them. It seemed to me that the food that had appealed to him recently, while certainly being good for him (fresh fruit), was not giving him the calories that he needed to gain weight. He seemed to get thinner every day, especially his back. Every vertebra was so prominent, every rib so pronounced, bulging the thin dry skin that covered his back.

Often he asked me for backrubs like the ones his nurses in the hospital gave him. I was so afraid I was going to bruise or even tear his delicate, silvery, cracking skin. He could tell in an instant that I was being cautious, and he yelled and pleaded for me please to rub harder. We had built up a routine after a few workouts. I rubbed on some lotion, worked it in very, very hard, and then ran to the bathroom, where a towel was soaking in hot, steaming bathwater, and quickly wrung it out—I had to do this part very fast or else the towel would cool down—and then ran to John lying on the bed and wrapped the towel around his back, the fog of the steam rising from it. I think now, as I remember those days, that this backrub and hot-towel race gave John the only prolonged times of physical ease and happiness. Unspoken, riveting pain produced by even slight movements made up the rest of his day. Many nights we'd spend a couple of hours, not just twenty minutes, going from backrub to hot towel to backrub.

And his hip bones stuck out two inches, with the skin at the sides and back hanging. His skin didn't seem to have the same consistency, the same color, as it used to, as it used to not only before he got sick but before he underwent the first treatment. His skin was so thin now. There was no muscle or fat underneath it to help round out the contours of the bones it covered. Even his man's hairy legs and arms looked feeble, as if the hair on them had decided to lie flat and become colorless. Nothing vibrant about those arms or legs anymore. So ill. And I kept hoping that if only John could eat starchy foods, if only they didn't turn his stomach, his skin would get its resiliency back. So I not only got tired of cutting up grapefruit halves, I also knew they were useless as far as putting any weight on John. But I couldn't bring myself to comment, to criticize what he ate, in effect to *nag* him to eat things that didn't appeal to him, to tell him he had to gain weight.

Not too long after he came home from the hospital after that first treatment, he began to ask me to leave him alone when he ate. Very often he had to spit in between bites, and the slow chewing and eventual swallowing embarrassed him. I wonder now if he threw away a lot of the food because he just couldn't stand it. It didn't occur to me then, and I wouldn't have asked him anyway. I respected him too much. Something so few people could see. That here was this terribly ill man, and except for my trying to make him as comfortable as possible I treated him as a normal, living man. And asking him if he'd finished his lunch, eaten every bite, would have turned my stomach if not his. I also know he would have been hurt and disappointed if I had checked up on him like that.

I only checked up on him once. He was going down to Kelley Drye for the first time since he'd been home from the hospital. He had on some new pants, also purchased by me at Gimbels, that must have been at least a size 44 waist, so that they could fit over his huge tumorous stomach, and he had on a Brooks shirt that was now so big around his thin neck that when he put his tie on and knotted it, it pulled the cloth of the collar around so much that it looked pleated, and over that he wore a navy-blue shetland pullover sweater, and over that his navy-blue blazer. This was not because he was cold—on the contrary, his cancer made him incredibly sensitive to heat—but these layers of clothing were camouflage, devised by him and me, to make him look filled out, to hide the painful thinness of his arms, back and shoulders. And then he lifted up his new briefcase that I'd given him for his partnership in the firm—it was so heavy for him, but he was determined to take it with him. On went the Rolex watch, which he hadn't worn since before his operation. It was so big for him that quickly I had to get out a pin and push in the sprockets and adjust the stainless-steel bracelet to its tightest size. I fastened it on him. It fit, but it weighed down his hand so. I'm off, he said. I begged him to take a cab when he mentioned he might walk down. I couldn't believe it, walk down thirty-five blocks, when just about everything tired him. I shut up when he told me he was going to walk, period. I gave him a kiss, I loved him so much, and he was out the door, and I heard the elevator doors closing.

I ran to the phone and called his friend Tom Davis,

whose office was right next to his, and told Tom to please call me when John got in to tell me he was all right, explaining that he had refused to take a cab and was walking down. And I told him not to let John know he was calling me because he'd get mad.

Tom called about forty-five minutes later. John had walked only a few blocks, had felt tired and had begun hailing cabs, but there hadn't been any for a long time, and that was what had taken him so long getting to the office. But he was there now and was fine, although Tom was shocked at how he looked, as everyone would be.

The news of John's arrival and his appearance traveled fast, and there were many, really most of the firm, who couldn't go in to see him, who knew their look of stunned disbelief would be read by John immediately. John knew and understood and was actually grateful that people didn't come in and gawk and tire him out. He also knew, as I found out later in the afternoon when he came home, that I had called Tom. And he told me, "Nini, don't you ever do that again. I mean it." His lips pressed together and there was fire in his eyes, and I knew he was damn, damn angry with me.

He was furious, and he went straight back to the bedroom to get out of those hot, hot clothes. I didn't even dare to go in to talk to him for at least an hour. I felt so ashamed, but I cared so much, I worried so much that he might not get there all right. I promised him and myself that I would never check up on him again, but to please forgive me this first time out.

It was a few days after that incident when I brought in his lunch tray and went out of the room while he ate and put the useless earphones back into their box and headed back out to Gimbels. Hell, nobody wants to hear this, least of all me, because it was a day really to be forgotten, but I went up the eight levels of escalators to the return desk, and they were more than surprised to see me again with another set of earphones to return for credit. Our bill, I thought, was going to take a wizard to figure out when it came in the mail with all the credits and purchases of earphones. Finally I was back with the saleswoman at the audio counter. She didn't believe they didn't work until she tried them herself. Oh, she said, yes, come to think of it, we have had some problems with these earphones. I told her about John, about the fact that he had to have these lightweight earphones and wouldn't she please sell me the display ones.

And I started feeling sick; all of a sudden my six-month pregnancy was making itself known. I felt dizzy and I just wanted to get this over with and get out of there. Other people were complaining that I'd gone ahead of them, that it was their turn for the saleswoman to help them. The saleswoman explained that I'd been there earlier and that this exchange would take only a moment and that she'd be with them in just a moment. The box was taped up, went into a bag with the sales slip stapled to the fold, and after signing yet another charge slip and putting the charge plate back into my bag, I walked back to the escalators. God, eight levels back down. I grabbed on to the black rubber railings as if they were the only reason I didn't fall. By the third floor I could feel that I was on the verge of crying. I was so tired. I didn't ever want to go into that store again.

When I got home, John was taking a nap. I knew he would be happy when he woke up to find I'd gotten a pair of earphones that worked, and he was. But before he tried them, he was going to take a shower. And then he would come out and put on the earphones and listen to WQXR for the rest of the day.

These showers were something that started up at Presbyterian. John said that the steaming water, like the steaming towels when I gave him a backrub, helped the pains in his back. But in his long hospital stays John hadn't realized how very much weight he'd lost, because the bathrooms had only shaving mirrors, not full-length ones, so he wasn't aware of how terribly much he'd changed. It wasn't until he got home and took a shower and saw himself before our mirrors that he knew, that he saw.

He was so frightened when he saw himself the first time. He called me into the bedroom. "Nini," he said, standing there dripping on the towel he'd tossed on the floor, looking down at his naked, wasted, flesh-hanging body, "did you know I'd lost so much weight?" There he was standing there with his huge, swollen, skin-taut stomach, like a Biafran child, and the rest of him stick-thin. "How much do you think I've lost, Nini?" And I lied, I would lie over and over again, because there was a tone in his voice that begged me not to tell him how really awful he looked, a tone that wanted to hear he was the same robust, sexy man, that he was the same husband I had always loved, as if he were scared a change in his looks would change the way I loved him.

So I lied, and it didn't even matter. "Well, Bunky," I answered, "of course you've lost weight. It's to be expected. After all, you've undergone major abdominal surgery and have had your first chemotherapy treatment. But don't worry, Bunk, it'll come back. I don't think you've really lost too much. You look the same to me, just a bit thinner. But I'll feed you well. You just tell me what you want and I'll make it. How about I go into the kitchen and whip up some *boeuf en gelée*?"

And how he laughed and grabbed me to him to hug me. He remembered that two summers before I'd spent two days making *boeuf en gelée* for a very fancy dinner party we gave. The day of the party I even kept running back and forth from school to spoon over more *gelée*, to make sure the *gelée* had jelled, and for some reason, the work that went into it, and my seriousness about doing it right, enchanted John. Also, he said it was the best thing he'd ever eaten, but more than that he loved the methodical, earnest way I went about making it.

When he came out of the shower, he had on a pair of pajamas Uncle Jack had sent him because John's no longer fit around his stomach. The bottoms had a drawstring waist, and the top was big enough to button over his stomach. He brought out some pillows for his back, along with my father's heavy book of the collected Sherlock Holmes mysteries, which John had asked if he could borrow, and he eased himself onto the couch, put on the earphones, closed his eyes briefly in bliss to the sound of one of his favorite tenor arias, and with great effort lifted the Sherlock Holmes book up over his stomach and began to read. He called out for some tea with honey, and when I returned with it, he smiled.

I headed back to the kitchen, but I sneaked a peek at him in the mirror that faces the living room. He was so happy, he was comfortable. It was such a strange life we were leading, because it was so different from our previous nine-to-five workdays, but I was happy. And even at that early stage of his quickly ravaging cancer, I looked down at my own stomach and believed John would see our child.

CHAPTER SIX

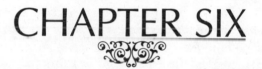

Dear Lizzie,

What a comforting, wonderful letter you wrote back to me. Everyone has been trying to be helpful, but no one has really understood—especially understood the aloneness of this experience for me. But you understand. I'm more convinced than ever that happy marriages are very rare—so rare in fact that yours and mine are perhaps even more spe-

*cial than we ever thought. It is because you and Woody
are so happy and are so perfect for each other that you
understand what sadness John's illness causes me.*

*. . . John is trying to strengthen up before the next 5-
day treatment, which starts this Sunday. And he tries
to get out for a walk in the park every day, and every
other day he's been going into the office for 3 or 4 hours.
However, recently his legs and feet have started to swell
because (his doctors tell him) the fluid the tumor produces is "shifting." (???) This means though that he
must keep his legs elevated, so walks and the office are
out for a while.*

*Yesterday was a big day which John met with good
grace, strength, and even humor! We went downtown to
a hair salon that specializes in fitting wigs for chemotherapy patients. I wasn't quite sure how this hair fall-
out was going to occur—I kind of expected clumps, I
guess—but it's really just like a dog or a cat shedding. It
is amazing how fast it happens once it starts, but John
now has a very natural wig, and he's quite pleased with
it—says he looks a hell of a lot better than Howard
Cosell!*

*Apparently we may see some results of the chemo-
therapy after this 2nd treatment instead of after the 3rd
as we were originally told. A decrease in the huge size of
his abdomen will show something is working.*

*I go up and down emotionally—John actually still can
do his wonderful cheer-up act for me. I find it hard
though to go about buying the crib, etc., without him.
Also making arrangements for two neighborhood husbands to take me to the hospital if I require a middle-of-
the-night trip is hard. So far looking forward to this
baby is good for me, but the thought of maybe having no
one to share those first steps, etc., with is one I try to
put away. It certainly is true that only one day at a*

time can be faced. And for all the heartache there really is joy and humor in each day.

It is so strange how different people have reacted to this. We have one set of friends, a couple, who are almost vulture-like in their wanting to know every latest detail and wanting to be in the middle of this. Really almost sick behavior, and it has shocked both me and John because it is so far beyond the simple offer of help when needed. It's gross overkill to the extent that one thinks they have latched on to us and this sadness to fulfill some private need. To my utter shock, Anne-Marie even tends toward this. She keeps telling me it's all right to cry and not to hold back. Hell, what does she think I do at 3 a.m. when I come out to the living room so John can't hear me? She just keeps saying it whenever I see her. So far the only people I can cry in front of are John and my mother, and I'd like to keep it that way. And yet there are other people who react perfectly and show so much dignity and strength in their words and actions that they are the ones who lift you up and make you realize you can cope. You are at the top of that group, and this lengthy discussion had as its purpose just that to tell you. Whenever you have one of those "worthless, I haven't accomplished anything" days, please remember your heartfelt letter to me eased my pain and helped me to become stronger—truly!

JSM said how much she loved seeing you and that you have licked the pneumonia. Please do wrap up warmly and don't overdo! Perhaps when you have time you could write and tell me about your apartment, the restaurants, etc., you and Woody have been to, the weather, exhibits you've seen and so forth. As I no longer go into school, I miss that contact of regular daily life.

*I think of you so often—stay well, and, again, thank
you for your perfect words and feelings.*

All love,
Nancy

As John began to withdraw more and more to the earphones and to his books, when the doctors suspended,
they hoped temporarily, his trips to the office and his brief
walks, he also withdrew further from me. I knew what it
was like to want to be alone myself—John had taken the
hint after my ectopic pregnancy to tread softly around me
during the few weeks of convalescence—so now, too, I felt
his moods should be respected. He knew I was there if he
wanted anything, but I was determined not to get on his
nerves, not to get in his way. I wrote more and more in my
diary, and my letters to Lizzie increased. When I went into
our room with the mail for him, I learned not to try to give
him a kiss or even pat his arm or leg as I put the mail on
the table beside him. If I did try he would shake his head,
look up at me with his pale face, which he didn't have to
shave anymore as no beard was growing in, his sparse
hair uncombed, and with a brutal look he'd say, "Don't,
Nini."

"Okay, John. I'll leave you alone. Is there anything
you'd like from the kitchen? No? Okay. Call me if you
want anything." And I'd softly close the bedroom door,
when actually I felt like slamming it, and walk quietly back
out to the living room to open the mail that had come for
me: notes dropped off by people at school, was there anything they could do? Then bills to be paid, sitting at the
dining-room table wondering how we were going to be
able to pay the doctors, the hospital bills, both John and I
feeling awkward and as if we hadn't planned for such a
disaster when his father paid a lot of the bills for us, then
thank-you notes to be written to those who'd dropped off

cakes and cookies they'd made for John—word had gotten
out that he liked chocolate-chip cookies.

On this particular morning I sat writing out checks to
Con Edison, New York Telephone, and I glanced out the
window and saw a raggedy, yelling stray of a man, an old
man, his white hair tied in a ponytail down his back, yelling at the people who passed him on the sidewalk and at
the cars and buses, too, shaking his fist with anger, and
my stomach turned as I remembered that I hadn't seen
him walking around the neighborhood recently. I had
passed him often enough walking up to Nightingale at
92nd Street in the mornings. One morning in fact I'd been
humming a song to myself and thinking about what I had
to do that day at school, and I hadn't been paying attention, I hadn't realized he was approaching me, otherwise I
would have quickened my stride and even stepped out
onto Madison Avenue to get around him as I'd done other
times, but I was too late for that. I looked up, and before I
knew it, he came rushing toward me, throwing his arms
and hands out stiff in front of him and into my face as if to
say "Boo!" He was shouting gibberish and glaring at me,
and I jumped between a couple of parked cars and out into
the street. Then he yelled so that I could understand him,
"Sure, run away"—mumble, mumble—"old man . . ."
Then, pointing his finger at me: "You, you!" He kept on
walking, still turning his head back to look at me every
couple of steps and to point and yell at me. My ankles
shook; I went back to the sidewalk and leaned against the
doorway of a locksmith shop and tried to breathe in and
out very slowly. And then I ran the rest of the way to
school.

And here he was today outside my window doing his
same stuff, and all I could think was, Why isn't it you?
Why don't you have cancer? You're useless human garbage. Why couldn't it have been you?

Naturally every day after that I managed to see him as I went back and forth from Mt. Sinai to visit John when he returned for his second treatment, and I learned that he went up to Mt. Sinai himself every morning as an outpatient to get his medication and so was walking back downtown from there when I saw him. Even more than the glassy-eyed, frail little old ladies and men wheeled by their attendants in their wheelchairs to get some air, just like a baby in a carriage—women and men of whom I'd think, Your time is up anyway, you're all ninety-nine and a half, why isn't it one of you instead of John?—this man, this white-haired ponytailed man, came to represent to me the unfairness of life. Why hadn't he ever been exposed to asbestos?

That damn asbestos. What a touchy subject. Taking Dr. Lisio's advice, I never did mention it to John but waited for him to initiate any conversation about it. The first time was one late afternoon a day or two after the operation when we were alone together in his room, and he turned and said, "I guess you know that what I've got was caused by asbestos?" I nodded, and he continued, "You know those jobs I took, I told you about some of them, the construction jobs, the 'no more heavy lifting' jobs," and he looked from me down to the sheet spread over his legs and shook his head. "Well, for two weeks I loaded and unloaded this asbestos sheeting on and off the trucks. They didn't have a fork-lift truck at this place, so what the men and I would do would be to lick our thumbs as we counted off these sheets and then heave a bunch of them onto the truck and they'd land with a bang." Oh, oh, I thought quietly to myself, *that's* why it's in his abdomen. Then he said, "I just wanted you to know, but also, Nini, well, I don't feel like talking about it, so I'm just asking you not to talk about it with me either, okay?"

So Dr. Lisio was right. It would be another six weeks

before John referred to it again with me; of course, with his doctors he had to talk about it all the time.

A couple of days before John went back into the hospital for his second treatment he had an appointment as an outpatient to have a scan in the Nuclear Medicine Department. He'd gone back one other time to his old floor to have more accumulated fluid produced by the tumor tapped off, and he'd gone up there by himself that time, but this day he was feeling a little shaky, so we went up together, and walking through the underground maze of hallways connecting all the buildings at the medical center, we finally found the Nuclear Medicine Department. The most memorable thing about that visit was the nurse behind the desk, who looked at my pregnant stomach when I got up to stretch as John and I sat there waiting and waiting for his name to be called, and yelled, "Get her out of here! There's a pregnant woman here!"

I looked at John, looked at the nurse; yes, she was talking about me. She rushed over, her rubber heels making a sucking noise on the linoleum floor, and put an arm around my shoulder. "My dear," she said, "I couldn't tell you were pregnant sitting down. You've got to leave. We never let pregnant women into this area of the department. Now if you go out that door and go down the hall, you'll see the opthalmology department. There're a couple of waiting rooms there. You wait in one of them, and I'll be sure your husband meets you after his scan."

She rushed back to her desk, and I raised my eyebrows and shrugged my shoulders at John, squeezed his hand as I stood before him and said I'd see him when he was finished. Jesus Christ, that's all I need, I thought, as I walked out of the doors and down the hall, kind of slowly at first and then walking faster, finally my walk breaking into a run, and the overhead fluorescent lighting glaring in my eyes—John's got cancer and now the baby's going to get it, too, or be deformed. Oh, shit.

I sat down in the empty children's waiting room, big colored balloons painted on the walls, red plastic couches and chairs. My face was flushed with heat. I got out of my coat and looked down at my tan corduroy jumper and patted my stomach, thinking, It just never stops, does it? Just never lets up. Once you're on a roll of disaster, don't expect anything to be easy, because as hard as it is to believe, it just keeps getting worse.

Not since the summer had I spent time thinking about and imagining what the baby would be like. Now I didn't have the time for it. Oh, I knew I had to take the special vitamin pill every day and drink milk and eat fruits and vegetables. I knew that the drugged comforts of alcohol and sleeping pills and tranquilizers were not allowed me, this as I watched the other members of our families gulping down a drink, reaching for a cigarette, taking a Valium. Whatever hold I had on my composure was due to writing in the diary and writing to Lizzie and knowing that I had to continue to eat, when eating then turned all of our stomachs—we just didn't have any appetites—because I had a baby growing inside me. So the vitamin pill and eating three meals a day were daily laws, but that was my extent of thinking about the baby. Now I looked down and thought, Oh, no, little baby, not you, too!

I'd already been reassured by Dr. Wiedel; in fact, he'd brought it up because he didn't want me to worry that the baby might have cancer, saying, "I don't know if you've been worrying about this or not, but I want to assure you that John and you could never have conceived unless he'd been perfectly healthy at the time. I just want you to know this so you won't spend time worrying about it." And with that I felt some relief that I could forget about the baby and go on with whatever needed to be done for John.

So the nurse's reaction to seeing me scared me. What have I done? I thought. I've had lunch, I haven't taken any drugs, I've taken every possible precaution, and *you're* telling me to get out of a potential high-radiation area? Could it be that I've exposed this child to a danger that will catch up with him or her twenty years from now?

I had nothing to read and there were no magazines, not even *Highlights* or a *Sesame Street* magazine, or even some books in the corner. I went across the hall to the other waiting room. Nothing there either. Nothing to do but sit and wait and think, think about what I avoided every day, think about the real possibility of losing John, that the treatments might not work, that I might be left alone to bring up the baby by myself. I dragged one of the chairs around in front of me, put my feet up on it and closed my eyes and willed myself to think about nothing, just nothing.

About an hour later John came in, walking slowly with his hands on his back, obviously in pain. He stood there looking down at me, his maroon running suit, the only clothes he felt comfortable in, pulled tight around his big stomach, and said, "Let's go. Yeah, I'm all finished. They did the scan. Jesus, lying on another steel table; I'd like to put one of those residents on that table. Goddam, it hurts."

We tried to retrace our steps and to find our way out of that Gustave Levy black box of a building, and as we slowly walked along, John said, "I got a nice compliment back there."

"Yes?" I asked. "Tell me about it."

"Well, they put me into a wheelchair to wheel me around to the CAT scan, and when we got there there was a gray-haired woman—at least what she had left of her hair was gray, you know, kind of like me, not much on top anymore—oh, about sixty-five years old I'd say, and she was sitting there in her wheelchair. Well, they wheeled me up right alongside her, and she looked over at me and said, 'My goodness, what a handsome young man you are!' " And John grinned his old aren't-I-the-sexiest-most-handsome-guy-in-the-world grin at me.

And I smiled and asked, "And what did you say to her?"

"Oh, I thanked her, sure, she was smiling at me so nicely, and then I said, too—I mean she looked even worse than I do—I said, 'Well, it doesn't really matter much anymore, does it?' And she nodded her head and said, 'Yes, I suppose you're right.' We talked about her children, who her doctors were here. I enjoyed talking with her. We both wished each other luck."

John paused and leaned against a wall—we finally could see the exit up ahead—and said, "Can you imagine anyone calling me handsome these days?" Then he gave a short laugh, but there were tears in his eyes.

I squeezed his hand and said, "I think you're handsome, Bunk."

And for the first time in weeks he held my hand, put an arm around my shoulder, and as we walked out into a darkening late afternoon on Fifth Avenue to get a cab home, he said, "I love you," and patted my head.

Don't think that it became any easier after that for John to talk about his cancer. For him, not talking about it, except in terms of when one treatment would end and another begin, was one of the ways he protected himself, that and continuing to wear his jogging suit. But at least we had our friendship back. I was no longer someone to be avoided; and lying in our bed together that night I could finally relax: we were allies, determined to remain very much the same married couple we were before we ever heard the words "mesothelioma" and "asbestos." Without saying much, mostly by gestures and looks in our eyes, we agreed, intuitively really, that whatever time was left would be spent as much as possible as we'd spent our married life.

John would not discuss his approaching death with me or anyone else (although I learned two years later from his mother that to a priest in the hospital John had said that he was not afraid of dying but that he was worried about what his death would do to me and his baby and his family). Perhaps because we were at times lifted by hope from the doctors that the next treatment might work, give a remission, we dared to ignore the possibility of his dying.

So when he went back in for his second course of chemotherapy treatments, he was almost buoyant, a sort of "Hell, the first treatment wasn't so bad, this one'll be a piece of cake" attitude. He was put in a different part of the hospital, in a much older wing, in a room by himself, with a big old color television and, best of all, a refrigerator! It was on the opposite side from his first room, so now he had a view of the other side of the black-box building; also, something nice, outside the window was a little balcony. But the room was dark, the paint dingy and peeling, the elevator in the building rarely worked; he loved it but it depressed the hell out of me. As he would lie on his side with a catheter inserted in his abdomen so that the fluid would drain off, this awful dark blood-colored fluid filling up a gallon glass jar on the floor and he or I making sure to call the nurse in time to have her remove it and bring a new jar in before the old one got too full, he would dictate shopping lists for me. Please bring tomorrow, Nini: orange juice, ginger ale, vanilla and chocolate ice cream in Dixie cups, lots of pears, and some brownies. And while he was talking, new jars for the fluid and new bottles of Adriamycin and other IV liquids were being brought in and the used ones taken away by the nurses. And it all seemed perfectly normal. John's old roommate had a

room on the other side of the hall, and one day we both
saw a very attractive woman go in to visit him. "Yup," he
told us later, "that was my ex-wife. Pretty decent of her to
come visit me. We didn't fight once!"

While John was in for that treatment I did things like go
to the dentist, the dentist I've seen since I was thirteen
years old. "How are you, Nancy? Oh, no, really? Hoping
to keep John alive to see the baby? Oh, my God." He and
the lovely Oriental hygienist were leaning over me, their
hands and instruments in and out of my mouth, as I told
them in between their fast-moving hands what had happened. I told it by rote now; only by being numb could I
talk about it so calmly. The last thing I wanted anybody to
do was to put his arms around me and try to comfort me
about something that was comfortless.

At least, though, I was steeled for meetings like that; of
course the dentist would ask how I was, and I would have
to tell him what had happened. What was worse was having a doorman tip his hat to you and say, "Bet it's a boy!"
as you walked by, or to get into a cab and have the driver
say "This your first? Bet you and your husband are real
excited," or to go into a store to buy baby furniture all by
myself. There was a store over on Amsterdam Avenue in
the nineties, Albee's, a family-owned and -run store, and I
went there one day with a list of things to buy. "A crib—
oh, the mattress is separate? Well, okay, if you say that's
the best one, sure. Oh, a bumper pad, hadn't thought of
that. Yes, the yellow one's fine. And a chest of drawers,
the one that can also be a changing table. And a carriage,
not a big one. Yes, it does make sense, this one that can be
removed from the frame to make a car bed, and the frame
folds up, too? The mattress comes with it, doesn't it?
Good. Do I want to bring my husband over to look at what
I've chosen? Well, yes, you're nice to offer, but he's in

the hospital. Yes, in the hospital. What does he have? Cancer."

I could feel it coming, I should have been prepared that this family-run store would be chatty, with a "Well, when's the baby due?" almost grandmotherly quality about it. I knew I had to be very courageous to go there by myself, but I hadn't anticipated that anyone would ask family-type questions. I thought I had anticipated everything: I had my list so that I could get in and out of there quickly, but it couldn't lock the door of curiosity. People just love to talk to an expectant mother. And why not? For everyone else it's a happy time, so of course a stranger would feel on safe ground talking and asking about it. And now that I was so obviously pregnant it was strangers' kind smiles that would make me sad, make my voice choke. The lady at the checkout counter in the supermarket must have wondered what she'd said wrong when I bit my lip and looked down, totally absorbed in counting out the money for her, when she asked, "When's your baby due? January? I could tell. My son and daughter-in-law are expecting their first in January, too. They've already painted the baby's room and have all the furniture ready. I told them I didn't believe in that, but, well, I'm just the superstitious type, I guess. I mean, what if something went wrong?"

And I, as I gave her the money, said, "I think I have exact change."

"Well, good luck," she said.

"Yes, thank you." I couldn't wait to get out of there; I didn't want to hear about other couples painting nurseries.

Also, I was starting to become scared, really scared. What was a life without John going to be like? How was I going to bring up a child by myself? One night in the apartment while John was still in Mt. Sinai I watched a television program about a woman doctor in Los Angeles who worked with premature babies. It showed her going in and out of her home, and at one point the camera panned on a lineup of photographs on her dresser; the one in the middle was of a young man, and she said that the hardest thing she'd had to adjust to in her life was the death of her husband when they were so young. That they'd had a happy marriage, and she wished they could have had a longer time together. I started to cry, just listening to her. She made it real. Yes, women do lose their husbands, they even die young. I'm going to be like her, I thought, and it scared me to think that I, too, would have a bureau full of photographs of my child and of John and that in twenty years a photograph of him would look dated, as dated as the photograph of this woman's husband looked to me. That woman made me face the possibility of becoming a widow.

I turned the television off and tried to read that morning's paper, but I kept raising my head and staring out the window. The news has nothing to do with me and my life, I thought, and I whispered, "I can't lose John now. I don't want to be alone." When, I thought, when are his chemotherapy treatments going to start to work? Seeing him in the hospital that day, trying not to mind the pain in his leg as he had to lie on one side so that the fluid could drain out of him—six quarts that day. And the IV in his arm. Those dear thin arms. "Oh, God," I finally yelled, "I want my Bunky back! I want him back the way he was, healthy, active." Impossible to sleep that night. I held Leo the cat in my lap, this dumb wonderful cat looking up at my face as he watched me cry, looking at me almost with concern.

Fortunately it was during this second treatment of John's that one of the social workers told me that the department of psychiatry, along with her department, was going to begin a pilot program of therapy for the spouses of those with cancer, and would I like to participate? I said yes, maybe so I could say how frightened I was of each day and of the future.

John came home from the hospital a couple of days later. The second treatment had made him feel much weaker than the first one. He was eating much more, which seemed a good sign, but along with the fatigue and weakness, I worried about his disorientedness. I told him three times one morning that I was going to the hospital to see the social worker and the psychiatrist who were going to be the leaders of the therapy group, and I told him when I would be back, but when I got home, he was wild-eyed. Where had I been? He'd been so worried. Oh, no, I thought, this is something new.

"I told you, Bunk," I said, "I told you before I left that I was going to the hospital." I practically yelled it; I felt I had to almost shake him in order to snap him out of this daze, that I had to get him back to reality.

And he looked at me, truly a little confused. "You did, Nini? Guess I just don't remember. I've been napping all morning, and when I woke up and called to you and you weren't here, I got scared. I forgot about your appointment. I'm sorry. Please don't worry about it."

There's only one good thing I can remember about the next couple of weeks, as the expected recovery or re-mission did not occur, and that is a letter John's younger brother, Vincent, wrote to him. John looked almost like his old self as he laughed when he read it. Vincent was writing him two or three times a week about cases he was working on in their father's law firm, about girl-friend problems, but this one was about how the city of Utica had built something downtown called the Tower of Hope.

TUESDAY, NOVEMBER 14, 1978
12:30 P.M.

Dear John,

*As I survey the City of Utica from my perch here on the
12th floor, the soft mist of this gray afternoon is blemished
by plenty of ugly structures, but the worst (at least psycho-
logically) is the "Tower of Hope." Perhaps you are not familiar with this wonder of architectural doodling. It is an
elongated concrete box-shaped tower with a clock on top.
The clock is not a mere timepiece, but also plays music. The
music it has been playing for the past two months is "My
Way" by F. Sinatra (also old blue eyes). Given the volume,
you could probably hear it in your apt. in NYC if you could
get the people in the A&P to be quiet for a minute.*

*I wouldn't really mind all this except that yesterday,
while walking past the base of the T of H, I read the plaque
secured there and learned the Tower is dedicated to that
Hope of Hopes, Bob (as in Road to Wherever). That's right.
In Utica there is a tower (costing about 50 g's) to "The
Spirit of Bob Hope."*

*Now I bet not even Kansas City or Indianapolis can top
that.*

Get well soon.

Vincent

John loved this letter, and I think one of the reasons is
that it was written after Vincent had visited him, after Vincent had seen for himself how ill John was, and yet he was
continuing to treat him like a normal human being. I don't
know how to explain that Vincent and his sisters were, at
the beginning, pretty much kept in the dark about John's
illness except that his parents surely thought they were
doing the best thing for their children and were sparing
them pain. But the consequences of this caught me off

guard only days after the operation when I called Vincent, telling him how John was and so on and chatting, and then I told him that we felt very lucky about the doctor at Mt. Sinai and hearing about his success with his treatments and that we'd be meeting with him next week and probably arrange for John to be transferred there. Vincent broke in and said, "Treatments?" And I said, "Yes, chemotherapy treatments." And with that Vincent said, "Chemotherapy?" And then I hesitated, not believing that he didn't know but then not wanting to be the one to tell him if he didn't know, that maybe his parents didn't want him to know, and I remember thinking, What do I do now? But Vincent broke the silence and my confusion by saying, "What's going on? Tell me." So I continued, "Yes, Vincent, chemotherapy. John has cancer." A "What?!" escaped from him. "But I'm his *brother!*" he said. "Do my sisters know?" he asked. "I don't know, Vincent."

From then on as the weeks passed and relations with our families became more strained, when discussions of second opinions and transfers to other hospitals almost undid John and me, Vincent became John's and my protector. When John mentioned that his parents' request that he call every day was getting on his nerves, Vincent told him not to worry, that he'd take care of it. Vincent was the one person who could glide back and forth from us to his parents to aunts and uncles to my parents and back again without letting himself be drawn into allying himself on anyone's side. The only side he was on was his brother's, so whenever he picked up on something even minutely annoying to John or causing him to become restless and impatient, Vincent would somehow be able to take care of it without making the person he was talking to angry, even when it was about things quite sensitive. One cousin was deeply religious, sort of a born-again Christian, and only Vincent could quietly indicate to him not to bring up his personal beliefs when he visited John again, and to John's aunt he could gently say that John probably was not going to listen to the positive-thinking cancer tapes she'd ordered from Texas that she wanted him to listen to, not that John didn't appreciate her going to the trouble to get them.

I remember John asked me to listen to them first. "What're they like, Nini? Are they anything I'd want to listen to?"

"I think they might help, John. There's certainly nothing in them that's going to bother you, and you might as well give them a chance. The guy who talks on them sounds sincere enough and certainly believes in what he's saying. So I don't know, John, but I'll leave them here in the drawer with the tape deck."

Vincent had the most extraordinary tact, and I don't know what John and I would have done without him. His loyalty to his brother was heroic. When his parents told his sister Mary Ellen that it might not be a good idea for her to travel from Utica to see John, that it might be too upsetting, I believe it was Vincent who told her to go ahead.

The saying that when one member of a family gets cancer, the whole family gets it as well is true. From the beginning determination of all of us to stick together and do whatever was best for John, all of us descended into whining and complaining, a hell of hurt feelings and arguments, as if we had to prove to each other or maybe to ourselves that each one of us was still in control, still in control in an uncontrollable horror in which we were powerless. Some felt the doctors treated them with brusqueness and impatience, but my only concern was how they treated John, for if they were patient with him and thorough in answering his questions, that was what was important.

In fact, I've wondered since about the concern and attentiveness and kindness of all his doctors and nurses.

Their supposed attitude of cool, unfeeling detachment did not apply to John, and I've tried to figure out why. Was it John's youth and humor that had some of these men and women work on his case twelve hours and more a day? Was it the rarity of his cancer in a man his age? I've decided that were it only a matter of John's cancer being a scientific puzzle, the staffs of both the hospitals easily could have remained aloof and heedless of our questions and not have taken the time required to respond with their always extensive and frank explanations. They were always smiling when they spoke to John, and often their daily visits would ramble until they realized they were late.

No, it wasn't just his disease or just his youth or our expecting our first baby; it was John. They all liked talking to him. That this did not extend to every family member must have hurt, but I found myself tuning out or even walking away when the family discussed how awful the doctors were to them. They were wonderful to John, and, even more important, John trusted and liked them. I was not going to have his confidence in them interfered with by complaints that Dr. Chahinian or one of the other doctors had passed someone in the hall with just a few words and then sped on his way. One thing that was so obvious about the Neoplastic Department at the hospital was that the doctors were more research-oriented, much more like scientists; what was important to them was their research and trying to discover new and different combinations of drugs for use in chemotherapy treatments for the different cancers. Not the bedside manner a doctor with an office practice would be expected to have.

John didn't have a new treatment scheduled for another week, but it was a comfort to me, as I worried about his increasing weakness, that should anything go wrong, he could be put back into the hospital immediately. And something did go wrong, something that neither of us had been warned might happen.

CHAPTER SEVEN

John was getting thinner each day and much weaker and was starting to throw up. He hardly ate at all and could barely move from one room to another without it exhausting him. Worse, he had spent practically the whole of the past weekend in our darkened bedroom—didn't even want to read the paper. He had watched part of the Dartmouth-Princeton football game on TV and told me later how he could barely look at those young men ("my size, not like the players on the big university teams or the pros"). It reminded me of the day he looked out his hospital-room window and saw the little St. Bernard's boys playing soccer in Central Park across the street and turned to me and said, "I can't look at them," and of another day when he was first home and had gone for a walk in the park and came back telling me that the eight-to-ten-year-old St. David's and Day School boys, who were playing in the grass oval behind the Metropolitan Museum, made him feel so sad and sick, "worse than seeing the runners up by the reservoir." Also now he couldn't stand watching the TV commercials during football games, especially the beer commercials showing people eating pizza "and having a good time."

I barely got outside that weekend except to the A&P. Only seven weeks or more until the baby was to be born, and I was so tired by then. How tired I will be, I thought, once the baby actually is here. I would have to get some help. I thought John might need a nurse, and I decided to ask Dr. Chahinian about it when John saw him on Tuesday. If only there had been some improvement instead of that continual decline. Each week was worse for him than the week before, which at the time seemed unbearable and more than he should have had to withstand. I worried that John had lost all hope and optimism. Oh, why did it have to be him? Now even the smallest improvement would have been welcome.

I had to try to remain strong for him as he had for me so much in the past. I had to keep myself from burdening him. One night as he and I were reading in bed I started to cry, and John asked, "What's wrong, Little One?"

"John, I'm so scared."

"Scared about what, Nini?"

His voice was so concerned, so tender; didn't he realize why I was scared? "I'm scared about you, John. I don't want to lose you, I can't. . . ."

John nodded his head; he had understood. He leaned on one arm and looked straight into my eyes, and quietly but with measured strength he said, "Don't worry, Nini, I'll make it to the spring. I promise you. I'll see the spring.

Now dry your eyes and give me a kiss like a good girl. There."

And while I tried to stop crying I said, "But that's not what they told me."

"Look, Little One, trust me, I'll see the spring." And then he started to cry and said, "Look, Nini, you've got to be strong for me. You've *got* to be my brave little shaver. I need you so much. So, please, Nini, please don't cry, 'cause it's making me cry. I love you, and you've just got to stand up straight and be strong for me. I know you can do it, you know why? 'Cause you're my Little One and because you've got guts."

"You think so, John?" I asked, Kleenex swabbing both our faces. "I'll be strong, John. You, you can count on me."

"There," he said, as he and I rocked back and forth, our heads resting next to each other, his hand smoothing back my hair, my hand on his cheek, "now doesn't that feel better? Now no more crying, okay?"

It hurt to think that nothing I could do or offer was strong enough to stop his tumor and suffering. Only the chemotherapy could do that, and he still had to undergo a third treatment before we would know what effect the Adriamycin and 5-Azacytidine were having on his meso-thelioma. Patience and faith and strength: those were the things I prayed for, for myself and for John.

On Monday, November 20, John went back to 6 North as an emergency in an ambulance. John had been sitting on the couch in the living room when the color drained out of his face in seconds. He said, "Nini, you'd better call an ambulance. I've got to get to the hospital. I don't know what's wrong with me."

I ran back to the telephone to call Keefe & Keefe. Yes, they could be there right away with an ambulance. To what hospital would they be taking him? Mt. Sinai? Well, that would be a hundred dollars payable immediately. A hundred dollars for ten blocks. Yes, a check was okay. Next I called John's Uncle Jack, who worked in midtown. Could he come up right away? It was an emergency.

Uncle Jack arrived barely ten minutes later as the ambulance arrived. He led them up to our apartment; I opened the door and saw the stretcher being rolled down the hall. They squeezed it in through the door and went right for John on the couch. "We've got to get him up there right away," they said.

John could barely breathe and he grimaced with pain as they put him on the stretcher as gently as possible. I took his hand as they wheeled him out. John called back to Uncle Jack, "You take care of Nancy, please, Uncle Jack." I protested, said I wanted to go with him. "No, my love, please follow with Uncle Jack. I'd prefer that." I nodded, and Uncle Jack put his arm around my shoulders as we watched the end of the stretcher go into the elevator.

We walked back to the apartment door and closed it behind us, and I cried out that same animal cry I had tried to stifle the day of his operation, although this day I couldn't and didn't even think about trying to stop. John couldn't hear me now. "Oh, my God, Uncle Jack, what's going to happen? What's going to happen?"

Uncle Jack had the best idea and a sensible one; he knew I was on the edge of hysteria. He explained that it would probably take some time for John to be treated in the emergency room and a while before he was put in a bed in 6 North. He suggested we go to a restaurant and have a bite of lunch. Did I know a place in the neighborhood? And the one that came to mind was a place on 96th Street and Madison Avenue, a place where my class in high school at Nightingale would sometimes go for a Coke.

The day was brilliantly sunny, even on November 20,

and as we walked up Madison Avenue, we were enclosed in our own world, which had no relation to the shoppers and walkers passing us. I guess to take my mind off my terror, Uncle Jack asked me about the little shops and boutiques that we passed. Weren't most of them pretty new, opened in the last few years? We got to the restaurant and found a private booth. I was shaking, and he suggested I have a drink. I was going to have an iced tea but decided the baby wouldn't be harmed forever if I had a beer, which I did. We ordered sandwiches, and this pause, this break before going to the hospital, was what I needed. When we left and walked the few more blocks to the hospital entrance and as we went up in the elevator to 6 North, my hand tightly gripping Uncle Jack's, I realized all the more his wisdom in stopping for that lunch, for having taken a few deep breaths before walking down that familiar hall and inquiring after John at the nurses' station.

The news came. John had been near death, his respiration was so poor, and he had been given oxygen immediately. There was so much internal bleeding that he had been in shock. He had had an immediate transfusion of four units of packed cells and blood, and an IV of glucose had been started right away. He'd had a close call, they told me, but he was doing much better now, and I could go in and see him.

That night I felt so inadequate. Why hadn't I recognized the signs of shock? I'd gone into shock myself when I'd had the ectopic pregnancy. Surely I should have been able to tell by John's color, the clamminess of his skin, that he was in danger that morning. What if he'd been too weak to tell me to get the ambulance, if he'd been asleep even? He would have died! Why hadn't anyone warned us that this could happen? Why hadn't they told us the symptoms to look for?

Then Dr. Chahinian told me the chemotherapy had not worked.

On Wednesday, John was given an injection of C-Parvum (immunotherapy), which they hoped would make the tumor stop bleeding. The plan was to get John strong enough so that they could start a new course of chemotherapy on him, using different drugs as soon as possible. This so the cancer would not spread to other parts of his body.

For most of that week I felt hopeless and without faith. Thanksgiving Day was so painful—me cutting turkey for him, feeding him a few bites, John dropping the bread roll. Vacant stare. Eyes at one point rolled up into his head. I shouted, "John! John! What is it? Stop! Look at me!" His eyes came back down. Scariest thing I'd ever seen. He had lost much more weight, and his legs and feet were so swollen. Then the bedsore. This was new. How much could he endure?

But more alertness returned. He asked for the TV. His knees, though, gave out from under him when he tried to get back into bed from the commode three feet away. An accident report was filled out. Vitamins and albumin intravenously. He had to drink Sustacal, a high-calorie drink. John asked me to bring some glasses from home and put them in the freezer to make the Sustacal as cold as possible. It tasted terrible to him, so we tried freezing it as well. It came out quite thick, almost like a milkshake. With a straw he managed to drink it.

One very happy thing: the baby started to kick one day while I was there, and I said, "Let me have you feel this," and I put his hand on my right side. Thank goodness the baby obliged.

John said, "Wow! That's something!" and smiled the biggest smile. He kept his hand there while I prodded the

baby to do more. John kept saying, "Don't aggravate it."
Then he moved his hand all over my stomach, but by then
"Rudy" was back asleep.

I felt I had nothing to be grateful for on Thanksgiving
except that John had not died; I wanted more, I wanted
him to get well. I wanted him to see and *enjoy* this baby, to
see him wheel the carriage, to see him give the baby a
bottle, to see him as Santa Claus at Christmas 1979. Please,
I asked, let John be given good times again.

Actually my faith and hope had returned. What hills
and valleys, as John would have said.

My Diary:

SUNDAY, NOVEMBER 26, 1978

*John moved away from Mr. Fernandez in Room 622
and all his relatives. John so happy to be moved into 620,
and he's near the bathroom and across from the nurses'
station.*

*Unfortunately, his stomach is larger. IV is out though,
but still problems with diarrhea and his bedsore. His color
looks better, and I think he is a little bit stronger.*

*He tells me how much strength looking at my picture
gives him, and before I leave, he asks me to turn it toward
him. He asks me if I love him like old days. I tell him I am
depending on him. I kiss him goodbye, and he says, "What
a good kiss, what a good kitty." When I left he was watching television and seemed so much happier and relaxed
being in a room with a quiet roommate who also has hardly
any visitors. John asks Mr. Walker if he likes to sing, to
sing at 3:00 in the morning. Poor Mr. Walker wasn't sure
what J. meant but answered, "No." J. said, "Well, we'll
get along fine then." J. still, thank goodness, still strong
enough to make a joke.*

MONDAY, NOVEMBER 27, 1978

John again says what a comfort it is to have me there each day.

Today I cut his fingernails and toenails, and he doesn't object. Also put Neutrogena cream on his feet and Liquiderm on his legs.

Another argument with his father re this second opinion business. He saw Dr. Lisio this morning and asked him what to do. Not so bad in itself except, again, it was done without our knowing. He calls and apologizes this p.m. and says he is going back to Utica tomorrow.

Actually it was a pretty good day. Dr. Orsini, a new doctor on the 6 North rotation, telling me, and me seeing, how much stronger John is and that no new fluid has been produced by the tumor because the immunotherapy seems to be working. Didn't think though that John would have another chemotherapy treatment for two to three weeks.

Later saw Dr. Chahinian and explained J's room change. He was amazed at the number of visitors Fernandez has and the length of time they stayed. I told Chahinian I didn't want to bother him, and he said, "You're not a bother." He is obviously very fond of John and me. John saying to his father that he was afraid that a second opinion might make Chahinian more cautious, less willing to take risks on him.

It was nice to be there while John had his lunch. Said he'd had a big breakfast so for me "not to be mad" if he didn't eat too much for lunch. I said of course not. I know he's trying his best to eat as much as he can. He also is lying on his side a lot more. He's trying so hard and is so determined. Even drinking those Frostees.

Dr. Orsini also seems to think that unless John has a relapse, he very well may be coming home this weekend. That sure is hard to believe but would be a miracle from a week ago today. Actually everything is a miracle from last

Monday. John is going to keep on living. I love him so much. He cannot leave me yet—I want to hear him sing again.

TUESDAY, NOVEMBER 28, 1978

Bunky looks much better today. Said that even though he was up all night, diarrhea problem has been cleared up. Dr. Orsini said that yes he is much better but "not to get too excited." John's mother calls and gives me the impression that Orsini told his father that John's stomach was going down and that the chemotherapy (?) was working. If anything, it's his immunotherapy injection that's working. They are really nuts, and Vincent Sr. hears nothing. He only wants to hear that John doesn't have cancer.

John tells me he thought of me a lot last night. I said I hoped good things, and he said oh yes. He apologizes for being so sleepy when I come to visit. He liked my most recent card to him very much. . . . Please, God, let him have some good days, months, where he is able to walk, feels good. Let him fight harder and harder every day, and make him show us that he is determined to survive, and finally, let his fight be victorious. He must see this baby, and he must have some healthy time to enjoy him/her.

WEDNESDAY, NOVEMBER 29, 1978

Good check-up with Dr. Uscher. He is on time at 8:30 a.m. and spends half hour talking with me about John. Says he'd already chosen a pediatrician, George Lazarus, and says for me to call him. As it turned out, Dr. Lazarus had to call Uscher, so he heard the story from him. When I spoke to him late today, I didn't have to explain anything. He very interested that John diagnosed so recently in September and that he'd been so active two weeks before. Said it sure showed how vulnerable we all are. Anyway, said he'd like me to make an appointment with his secretary to meet him. Very nice. He said he and Uscher were residents together and had spent many 2 a.m.'s together, when I told him that Uscher had told me what a great guy he is. He said Uscher had told him that I was one of his very special patients.

John was asleep when I arrived today but woke up. I stayed while he ate lunch (all of it!). He told me that he looked at my picture a lot last night. I asked him what he wanted for Christmas, and he said, "Nothing." I said, "except the Little One." He said, "That's right." And I said, "And you're all I want for Christmas too."

Before I left he had the tap put in him for two hours of paracentesis. Then he would get his immunotherapy injection. John tells me that tomorrow they will start him on four days of the new chemotherapy.

I get confusion cleared up with Dr. Orsini re "good news." When John's mother talks to him, he tells her John "is stable and much better than when he came in and that it is now in the hands of God and the treatments." Orsini told me he'd told Vincent, John's father, that he "didn't think John would die," that John "would be home for Christmas," and that John's hemoglobin count had been good for five consecutive days.

The news does get better every day, but I can't allow myself the joy of abandoning myself to celebration and hopes and prayers fulfilled. John again tells me, "Life by the yard is hard; life by the inch is a cinch." I tell him he's covered a lot of inches this past week.

His face, abdomen and feet look so much better. Thank you, God, for these very real improvements. (Found a lucky penny in the 6 North phone booth today.)

THURSDAY, NOVEMBER 30, 1978

John awake when I arrived. He eats all of his lunch

(franks and beans and two slices of toast that his nurse Kit makes for him) and then eats the baked apple his Aunt Helen and Esther bring in for him.

He had his C-Parvum injection yesterday and by today the catheter for the paracentesis. Swelling in his legs and feet is much less, and for the first time, I saw him stand by himself and also bring his legs up over the side of the bed by himself instead of my having to lift them up for him. He smiles when I fix his pillow and say "Bum de bum." When I ask him if he's anxious to come home, he says, "Oh, Nini," and a look crosses his face that says that's all he wants in the world. He pulls out the mirror that belongs to the bed table, and says, "Yucch." I say, "Don't you think your beard looks snazzy?" He says, "Well, at least my cheeks have filled out a little." And then he blows out his cheeks like a chipmunk. After a while he says, "Well, enough of this," and puts the mirror back. . . . He wants to know when my next "class" is, his way of referring to the pilot therapy group I'm in for wives/husbands of cancer patients. He asks me what his bedsore looks like, and I tell him that he must stay on his side or else it will get worse.

Letter from Silent Unity, a gentle religious organization in Missouri that has a twenty-four-hour switchboard, and an affirmation: "My heart sings a song of praise! John is healed, praise God, John is healed!" Also, "You will forget your misery; you will remember it as waters that have passed away." Please let it all be true. Strengthen my faith, God, and do not let it falter.

FRIDAY, DECEMBER 1, 1978

In the morning at 10:30 I call the nurses' station and get Mr. Foote. He tells me that John's been moved back into 622A, Fernandez' spot. Obviously, Fernandez has died. I then try to reach Esther and Helen so they won't panic when they don't see John in 620. I couldn't reach them, as they'd already left. Mr. Foote also tells me John's blood glucose is down, which I later find out means that the tumor is producing insulin. I then call Karen Chamberlin, Chahinian's assistant, and ask when J.'s new chemotherapy will start and if this low blood glucose is corrected by blood units. No, she says, corrected by intravenous glucose. So that's it. She then tells me that Chahinian just found out about this condition and that she didn't think John would have any chemotherapy until next week. She also said not to worry about his care at home, as they'd probably transfer him off 6N after the chemotherapy onto another floor and would not send him home until he was well enough to function at home. I told her that John's mother would move in, having been a registered nurse, and that I'd been making inquiries about home care, and that maybe with John's mother's help we could swing it.

I get up there at 3:00 p.m. after Esther and Helen have left and am greeted by John's favorite nurse, Kit, who says, "John's doing great, and we've just gotten such good news. The test for the low blood glucose was done again, and it was normal. The first one was a mistake." John is so happy and tells me to call Esther with the news. Before that, though, John is sitting in his chair (!), and Kit makes his bed. Then Kit helps him out of the chair, and he walks by himself to the bed! He sits down on the edge, leans back, and she lifts his legs up. Now that is progress.

Lousy call to Croton to tell Esther news of test: I am told she can't come to the phone, that the result of the test is unimportant, and that Esther and Vincent are the only ones who are important. I cry when I hang up, and poor Bunky tells me to "sit in that chair for five minutes, relax, and then come give me a kiss."

I then go to my therapy group, and the young man is there—Pete—who is thirty-three. A big help as he has gone through parent problems (not in-laws—maybe his wife's parents aren't around) and understands. He tells me the baby will save my sanity as his son saved his, even though, as he said, a child added more logistical problems to his life: his care while he was at work and his wife was in the hospital.

Mrs. Levison, another member of the group, mentions that she worries I am trying to be too strong, and Dr. Brunswick nods his head.

I then go see Bunky and cut up his pork chop. He asks me if I love him, and I ask him if he loves me. He says maybe a week after the chemotherapy he can go home. I tell him how helpful his mother will be and that I am finding out about hospital bed, commode, etc., so that "you won't feel you have to walk to the bathroom." He says, "Let's see. I may not need them; I may be able to do it on my own." Before I left for the group, I told John that he'd done more and progressed more in the time I was there with him (the sitting in the chair, etc.) than all of the previous days. I tell him I probably won't be in tomorrow, and I tell him about my plan to make fruit cakes. He says fine, and I ask if I can call him; he says yes.

He tells me my strength is so necessary for him. He tells me, "I thought a lot about our baby last night, and I looked at your picture a lot." I tell him how proud I am of his fighting and that I depend on it for me and for Bunky #2. I tell him how much I need him.

Earlier I see Dr. Chahinian, who tells me, and then John, that on Monday, if John's urine is all right, he will give John a new one-day injection of chemotherapy. Poor Dr. C.'s face falls when I tell him, as answer to his question, that I've got six weeks at least left of pregnancy. He says, "I thought you said the baby would be born in December." I say the obstetrician says it is possible, but that I'm sure it will be January. Dr. C. tells me that this chemo-

therapy often has a side effect on the kidneys, which is why he must make sure John's are working perfectly before he gives him the treatment.

John very happy that it's just a one-day treatment. Says, "Well, that's good news!"

John loves me so much. I am secure in that and have no regrets. There is nothing I feel I must ask his forgiveness for. I am so lucky to have had this marriage. I mustn't let the loss of it and him make me bitter. All that is important is to be strong and happy for Bunky during these last days/ weeks. He just must not die in pain. And maybe he'll succeed in saying "Up yours" by living! Please, God, help me through these agonizing days and protect John and me and the baby. My love enfolds John tonight.

DECEMBER 1, 1978

Dear Lizzie,

. . . Your letters give me so much to think about, so uncannily reiterate private philosophies of my own, and give me the quiet strong confidence I need to go on. I want very much to reply confidently to your thoughts about God, that good behavior does not apparently mean freedom from tragedy, etc., but my mind is too firmly channeled into surviving the daily petty details of getting to and from the hospital to do it yet. But I look forward to the time when I can.

. . . As John and I had so hoped he'd be one of the good statistics regarding the effectiveness of the chemotherapy, it was a real blow to find out that was not to be. Days are filled now with monitoring of red cell counts, white cell counts, hemoglobin, blood glucose levels, etc. The immediate necessity is to get the tumor to stop bleeding so that they can try him on a new chemotherapy as fast as possible. The reason for this is that the one thing he has had in his favor is that the cancer hasn't spread to other parts of his body, and for

this to continue, he must get back on regular chemotherapy treatments right away. Unfortunately, his blood must be in good shape before they can do this.

Things have at least stabilized to a degree where I now call the nurses' station to find out how he is and not whether he's still alive! One really gets sort of a gallows humor after a while which is hard to explain and probably shocking to others.

How perceptive you are about people: Anne-Marie, Ellen. I really don't think, Lizzie, that my trusting nature in friendships comes about because I've got a generous, all-loving heart; I think it's because I'm dumb and just don't see others' ulterior motives and therefore am shocked when they appear with such strength that I can't avoid acknowledging this side of them. John's attitude about people has also helped—so often I've said how I can't stand one of his obnoxious friends or the wife of one of the partners or somebody, and he'll always point out how futile that kind of thinking is and show me their good points. This is not to say at all that he is some all-forgiving saint, but he just doesn't waste his energies on dwelling on peoples' faults and how they might affect him. Sometimes I've said to him that that attitude means he lives unrealistically and almost superficially, but I think ultimately he's right. So I try to copy him. What a ramble this is! Actually, as you predicted, Anne-Marie has been recently so terribly thoughtful, dropping off casseroles, etc., here so that I can just put dinner in the oven after a day at the hospital. It really has been a godsend. Patsy too has been incredible, leaving food with the doorman, inviting me out, etc. The people though who understand are those who've lost a close relative to cancer. They know how painful it is to watch the disintegration of someone you love. For instance, my marvelous obstetrician, Dr. Uscher, lost his mother to cancer, and his father died as well, in one year about two years ago when he was thirty-

five. He understands the realities of planning for a hospital bed in the home, etc. You won't believe his most recent thoughtfulness—he's already got the pediatrician for the baby and has explained the whole story to him and has arranged for me to meet him. I meet him next week and from his voice on the phone, he sounds adorable. And he's thirty-two years old. He certainly is a contemporary and will understand if I bother him with worries about fevers, eating habits, etc. of the baby.

I also was able to change my childbirth classes from the Wednesday "couples" night to Thursday afternoons. Except for the possibility of one husband who's a teacher and would be free at that time of day, it will be just five other women and me—in other words, no lovey-dovey cuddling garbage going on while I sit there alone. So many have offered to be in the labor room (and even delivery room) with me timing breaths, etc. I've tried to explain to these friends that if it can't be John, I don't want anybody there who knows him. It's going to be a rough emotional experience as it is, and I don't want anyone "taking John's place." If anyone helps me, I want a professional person on the hospital staff whom I've never met before. Also I've explained that I am going to these classes on Dr. U.'s suggestion only to learn what to expect. We both agree that this is not the time for me to prove I can withstand pain. And amazingly these women I know are shocked, saying that I'll miss such a "beautiful experience" if I'm not fully without painkillers. Shit. I figure Dr. Uscher is going to want to make this the easiest possible time for me, physically and emotionally, so I'm leaving everything in his hands. I also find it a little presumptuous for me or these friends to think that we know more about "birthin' babies" than an obstetrician who's delivered hundreds.

But to answer your question, yes, the pregnancy is fine and going well. I do get tired and out of breath easily but it's such a small price to pay for something you know I've dreamed of and wanted so much. People ask if all the kicking doesn't annoy me—are they kidding? This baby could do anything, and I'd be thrilled. All of which proves I'll be a rotten mother because I'll spoil the child outrageously! Well, at least this experience with John has gotten me over worrying what people think of me!

One last bit which may qualify me for sainthood: John's mother will move in with us when he comes home. She was an RN and really can take care of him, and we just can't afford the $90-a-day 24-hour care he will need. So I have no choice—I'm trapped—and I need her services. Pray it goes smoothly. Re cigarettes—I actually haven't had one although I am practically in the laps of those who do smoke. I've been dying for one so much even though it's been over a year since I quit. I wish I could tell you the desire for one goes away. . . . Keep it up though, Lizzie, you won't regret it. I just hope that after the baby's born I don't go back to it! . . .

All my love to you and Woody,

Nancy

My Diary:

SATURDAY, DECEMBER 2, 1978

God is still working for Bunky: good report from his nurse on the phone this morning ("He's eating more than enough and has been sitting in his chair") and from John when I called at 8:30 p.m. Voice sounds strong. I told him I would be up in the morning and that Dad would be coming with me. He said fine. I asked him if he'd seen Aunt Linuccia, and he said yes.

A day that refreshed my spirits: nice walk down Madison with Mom. Go into Paper East store and buy small presents for Gregory, Carolyn Clark's little boy, to open during the

baby shower, including a snowman in "snow ball," where the
flakes float in the water. Then to Leo's on 78th Street for
lunch: a ham and cheese omelet and a glass of wine. Then in to
Glad Rags but nothing there for my nieces, Stacey and Van-
essa, that exactly matches items on their Christmas list. Then
walk back up 5th to Mom's apartment, where she waters her
plants, and we have a cup of tea. So nice to be out of Apt. 2C
and 6 North for a day. I try not to feel too guilty or think I've
"abandoned" Bunky. So nice after yesterday's upsetting call to
Croton not to have to be the one who always understands and
nods head in agreement. A relief.

Earlier in the day Dad brought up New Yorker poster
that he framed for the baby's room. Was John's and my
anniversary present. Will tell John about it tomorrow. He'll
be thrilled, as he's wanted it for a long time. Then Dad came
back for dinner of leg of lamb. We all had a very good time—
I really enjoyed it. He certainly is a big help to have around
these days.

I can't wait to see John tomorrow. I ask J. how his day
was, and he says either "Nothing to shout about" or "Not
bad under the circumstances." I forget. I tell him I miss
him. He says, "I love you" and "Sleep well tonight, nighty-
night."

Is there a chance, God, with every positive thought and
prayer, that the chemotherapy shot may work? May I have
him a little bit longer? There is no life without him. Please,
please God.

SUNDAY, DECEMBER 3, 1978

Dad and I walk up to the hospital and get there by 11:00.
Dad comes in to see John after I've told John about Dad's
giving us the New Yorker poster for our anniversary. It's

*the first time my father's seen him in the hospital, as John
has wanted so very few visitors. John says, "Hello, Dick,"
and reaches over, even though he's lying on his side with his
back to the door, and shakes hands. He thanks Dad for the
poster, saying, "I've always admired it." John then says
he'd really like to snooze, so Dad and I go to the lounge. A
little later the nurse comes in and asks for Nancy and says
John said I could come in. I go back in. John tells me he
shaved yesterday for Aunt Linuccia, and that he sits in the
chair a lot. I tell him how proud I was to see him walk from
the chair to the bed. John says, "That's nothing." He says
he must get his exercise.*

*He then wants to go back to sleep. I go to the lounge and
then back to his room to sit quietly while he sleeps. I keep
saying, "He is healed, John is healed, praise God, John is
healed," while staring right at his back, willing that it be so.
John asks me how his bedsore is and says Dr. Hart says it is
healing. "This is the important thing now," he says, "to
get this sore to heal." He asks how much home-nurse help
is. "I'm going to need someone, my mother isn't strong
enough." I tell him about one of the social workers offering
to find out about our eligibility for Cancer Care and my
calling other places she's recommended. I tell him not to
worry as his major medical will cover it. He says he can't
wait to get out of there and to come home.*

*I ask him what he meant when he said a couple of
days ago that he'd spent a lot of time thinking about the
baby. He says, "I was wondering what kind of baby it
will be." I say, "I'm sure it will be a cute baby and a
smart baby." He nods his head. I tell him I miss seeing his
lower lip stick out, and he does it, and I say I needed to see
that. I also say I look forward to hearing him sing his songs
soon. I kiss his eyelids and hold his head. He says, "I love
you, Nini," and I tell him I love him and will call him
tonight.*

I call. Urine test results "inconclusive," but John says doctors think they'll go ahead on chemotherapy injection but that Dr. Chahinian will decide tomorrow. John says, "It is very confusing." He says he's in the middle of a heat lamp treatment. We say goodnight, and he says, "We'll see you, beuutiful."

I feel so blue all day. Angry at myself for wanting to get out of there today, not even to help him with lunch even though it was on its way. I felt I couldn't stand to be there much longer. Just feel crushed. To lose this dear man, this wonderful husband. How much is he required to endure? Other cancer patients get remissions, get to lead fairly normal and active lives between treatments for a while, but not John. It is too unfair. I feel there are only days left—not even weeks. I keep asking myself, "How can I live without him?"

Although depressed, Mom sends me off to bed happily by letting me open her shower present, a beautiful English wool carriage robe in Dress Stewart pattern from Bergdorf's. "Nothing is too good for my grandchild." I must remember the joy of the new life that John has given me that is coming my way. I must remember this blessing and thank God and dear Bunky for making this dream come true. As I said to myself the day of his operation, "I put my right hand in God's and John's other hand in God's and John in God's protection and care, as He will look out for us—the three of us—Mommy, Daddy and Baby."

MONDAY, DECEMBER 4, 1978

Esther and Linuccia in to see John and then me at apartment. I cannot go to hospital today—too much a flood of tears. Esther incredibly understanding and telling me that a man friend—never asked who it was—had told her to tell

*me that I have a life ahead of me and that I may think now
that no one can replace John, but that I must accept the
happiness that life will give me.*

*A wonderful introductory chat with George Lazarus.
What a comfort. He assures me the baby will be completely
healthy and normal, as the pregnancy has been so uncompli-
cated. He says Dr. Uscher plans to be with me the whole
time if I let him and that they want to get me and the baby
out of the hospital as soon as possible, so that "he or she can
meet his or her father." As I leave the office, he tells me he
feels he's known me his whole life and gives me a hug.*

*When Esther and Linuccia return from seeing John, Esther
tells me John is on Compazine and getting intravenous something to flush out his kidneys. By the time I call him at 8:00
p.m. (he answers after one ring), John tells me the chemotherapy (platinum and Adriamycin) is over and they are "now
just flushing me out" with the intravenous. When he answered the phone, he said, "Hi, Nini. I miss you." I say, "I
hear you're hooked up." And then John says that the chemotherapy is now over. He asks, "How are you?" I say, "I'm
fine." He says, "I'll see you tomorrow." I say, "I'll tell you
about the pediatrician tomorrow." He says, "Fine." Then: "I
love you, Little One, I love you very much. Take care."*

*Earlier I call Karen Chamberlin, Dr. C.'s assistant, re
autopsy, that I want to give permission when the time
comes but can I do it over the phone, that I don't want to
sign a paper in that hospital after he's died, and she later
tells me how grateful Chahinian is, and also that verbal
consent is enough, and that they all can't get over how
strong and realistic I am being. Earlier I suggest to her, too,
that they even give John a sugar-water injection because he
is so low and frustrated waiting for something to happen
after waiting three days for test results. Karen says that's a
good idea (!) and that she'll tell Chahinian. When she calls*

back later, she tells me John either is on the chemotherapy or is about to start it "imminently."

Please, God, let Bunky see his Bunky #2, whether it's a girl "Bunky" or a boy "Bunky."

Also, I called Mary Lehman at Kelley Drye today to make sure that I have the legal right re the autopsy and the memorial service. Mary says yes.

I look forward so much to seeing this baby. How happy we will be. I look forward to placing this dear creature in John's arms. May John and I please be granted that?

TUESDAY, DECEMBER 5, 1978

. . . Am up to 6 North by 11:05. John looks awful to me— no color at all. But little swelling, and his stomach almost seems flat.

He tells me how pretty I look and says, "I look forward to coming home and chasing you around the apartment." He says he thinks he'll be home in two or three days. He asks, "What's Leo up to?" I say, "Nothing much," and start to cry a bit. He says, "Nini, what's wrong?" in a worried voice. I say, "You are so brave." At that moment, Jane, the Hawaiian nurse, comes in to check his IV, and John says, "No, here's the brave one, my nurse." She leaves.

I tell him about Dr. Lazarus and give him his card, telling him that Dr. Lazarus said to call anytime.

John says he "overdid" last night: threw up. He says for me to come back tomorrow. I ask him if he wants to talk. That he can call and talk to me anytime. He nods. He says how pretty I look, pats his hand on my hair. He says, "Goodbye, Nini."

Esther calls at 2:30 to say Dr. Jacobs said to give John two or three days to see how this treatment works.

John: "I had a bad day yesterday. Tomorrow will be better."

WEDNESDAY, DECEMBER 6, 1978

Writing in here is saving my sanity, I think. It is a very nice way to end each day. I just wish I could remember even more the verbatim conversations with John.

I spoke to him this morning and told him that I wouldn't be in because I'd be resting up for the baby shower they were giving for me tonight. Then later conversations with Dr. Jacobs and Karen Chamberlin, Charlotte, Monsignor Wilders at St. Thomas More, Mary Lehman, John Callagy and his wife, Molly, Jack Garraty, all lawyers at Kelley Drye, and Esther.

Call John before I leave for the shower. I tell him I love him. He says for me to have a good time and tells me he loves me.

Lovely shower. I'm so glad I went. I actually got through it without crying. Lovely food, flowers, everything. And the most beautiful presents and cards.

THURSDAY, DECEMBER 7, 1978

I said to Mom about a week ago that I would know Bunky was better when he called me. Tonight he called! I tried to reach him at about 8:00 p.m. and let the phone ring six times. I then hung up, thinking that he was asleep. At 8:30 he calls me—said he couldn't reach the phone before. How am I? I tell him what a nice surprise his call is. He asks if I'd tried to reach him, and I say yes. He says, "I thought it was you." I tell him I'd forgotten to leave him the twenty bucks for the TV. I figured he'd run out of money. He said not to worry, to bring it tomorrow. I tell him I have a good letter from Vincent Jr. and will bring it tomorrow. He says fine. Finally I tell him Dr. Lazarus called wanting to know if he would like to meet him. I tell Bunky I told Dr. L. I would ask. Bunky says, "Isn't that nice. Tell him not to make a special trip, but if he's in the neighborhood, that would be fine." John then asks, *"When will you be up tomorrow, Nini?"* And I say at 11:00 and then also before or after my therapy group. He says, *"Good. See you tomorrow then, Nini. I love you."* I say, *"I love you, Bunky. Nighty-night."*

So much better than visit earlier in the day when I bring up Junel's quilt, Martha Rooney's handknit sweater and Susie Heller's blue-striped shirt and overalls. All of which he loved, but seemed so weak. When I asked what I could do for him, he said, *"Just be kind to me, Nini."* I said, *"Of course I'll be kind."* Left feeling very blue but happy that I'd held his hand. We both depend on our kiss hello and kiss goodbye . . . even if I do have to lower the rail on his bed, it doesn't seem to embarrass him. Dr. Lazarus is lucky to be meeting him—there is no finer man in the world.

Bad time at childbirth class. All the husbands were there, which the instructor had told me in advance wouldn't be the case. I told her I would not be coming back. Awful lack of understanding and compassion: she said once John had died I'd be welcome to rejoin the class. It made me feel she was talking about the death of a laboratory animal, not a man. Tell Dr. Lazarus about it when he calls. Dr. Lazarus also tells me he had lunch with Dr. Wiedel and relayed how wonderful I think he is. Dr. L. said, *"I told him you have excellent taste in doctors."*

It gives me confidence to know that Dr. Lazarus, who doesn't even really know me, is so anxious to be of help to me and John. His saying, *"I've thought of nothing else all week."* So many are there willing to help me. I must remember that.

Take cab ride home from childbirth class. Driver says, *"How was your day?"* I say, *"Don't ask."* He says, *"Oh, you can tell me your problems."* I say, *"You wouldn't want to hear this one."* He says, *"Try me. Unburden yourself."* I tell him, *"I'm a month away from having our first baby, and my husband is dying of cancer." He gulps and asks, "Is it terminal? Is there any hope?" I say, "No, there's no hope." He very quiet and then tells me that ever since he was at Anzio during WWII and mines blew up 300 feet away from him, killing many of his buddies, that "every day is a plus." He says he's been divorced twice, but he tells me that happiness does come again. I tell him that that is what my husband's doctors have told me. He says it's true. I start to get out my money, and he says, "This one's on me." I tell him, "I'll never forget this, Mr. Sugarman" (that really was his name!). He says, "Just let me see you smile." I try and then get out of the cab. There really are nice people left. I must remember that.*

Sleep tight tonight, Bunky. . . . God is going to take care of us both.

FRIDAY, DECEMBER 8, 1978

Because today was such a good day—good 45-minute visit with John this morning when I read him Vincent's letters, etc., good therapy-group session, and good visits with John before and after—I don't feel the need to write in here so much tonight. I think I can go to sleep peacefully, happily, and with some hope tonight.

SATURDAY, DECEMBER 9, 1978

Vincent Jr. arrives at around noon. Calls from Tappan Zee Bridge to say he'll be late. Terrible rain.

When he arrives, fix lunch and then we go up to John, who's just had a visit from Carolyn Clark, Esther and Linuccia, so he asks that we come back later in the afternoon. (Carolyn had brought him the flowers from the shower!)

Vincent and I then take bus to Tiffany's, where he buys two lovely hair combs for his girlfriend for Christmas. We then take bus back uptown, have coffee and tea and cookies and then take bus back up to John at about 4:30 p.m. Stay until 8:00 p.m. We get there just as Dr. Lazarus is leaving John's room. He stands out in the hall and talks for a long time with Vincent and me, telling us what a special man John is and confirming again that my pregnancy is going normally. Later when I go out to phone for John's TV service, Lazarus comes out of conference room. He'd spoken, I guess, to one of the doctors, who told him probably about John's case, maybe showed him John's chart.

Vincent helps John stand up! Then John sits on edge of bed for a while. Vincent helps move, carry, John when the nurse remakes John's bed.

Vincent and I leave at 8:00 and by then it's snowing. We eat at Adam's Son. Vincent seems to think John is better— encouraged by the absence of swelling in his legs and feet. I pray he may be right. Again, I tell myself I must "have confidence in God's promise."

SUNDAY, DECEMBER 10, 1978

Up to see John at 3:15 p.m. and stay until 5:00. We watch the end of Davis Cup Finals (McEnroe wins) and listen to Pavarotti tape.

A "renewal of life"—a phrase taken from Dr. Kirkland's Dial-a-Prayer today; I seem to have to call it when I wake up and when I go to sleep—is going to occur in John. I love him so much, and I know God is protecting us. This week I believe we will see a miracle; I believe we will see a beginning of the return to health I so desperately pray for in John; I believe John will be husband and father for many years. He is going to be truly healed.

MONDAY, DECEMBER 11, 1978

I pray I can believe the cautious news from Dr. Jacobs today:

1) *Platinum chemotherapy seems to have affected tumor positively. John had a sonogram this morning because Dr. Jacobs said they could not feel the tumor. Perhaps could this mean that the tumor has decreased in size? Jacobs said they could feel only fluid.*

2) *John's tumor is no longer bleeding internally as his blood counts are good.*

3) *Only tap for comfort, so no need now as fluid has not reaccumulated. This too, hopefully, because of platinum chemotherapy.*

4) *He does not think Chahinian will give John another immunotherapy injection this week (they'd skipped last week), but, of course, he said that is up to Dr. C.*

5) *They believe they may use a drug on John not previously used on humans in order to stop the tumor from consuming John's glucose. He said the drug would fool the tumor—that the tumor would think it was glucose—the result being that John and not the tumor would regain the benefits and nutrition from the glucose in his body. He said Chahinian would make up his mind in the next couple of days about whether or not to use the drug on John. Jacobs said they would not use it if the potential harm seemed too great—had to weigh benefits/harm very carefully before making a decision. Apparently, though, drug has been successful in this problem but told me not to get my hopes up. Said they'd have to obtain drug from manufacturer or NCI perhaps, but it is not at Mt. Sinai.*

Results of sonogram should be in by tomorrow. I hope Jacobs was not too optimistic.

I believe *the results will be good.* I believe *they will decide to use this new drug to correct John's glucose, and I* believe *the drug will work.* I believe *the platinum chemotherapy is the therapy that will give John a remission and years of life.* I believe *John will recover his strength and will be able to work at home.* I truly believe *God is protect-*

*ing us and accomplishing healing for John. I believe I will
hear more good news tomorrow.*

TUESDAY, DECEMBER 12, 1978

*John: "I may not show it or say it, but I really appreciate
seeing you every day."*

*An exhausting day with touches of hope that I'm not sure
I can latch on to or not:*

*Jacobs in with me and John; says Dr. Holland has ordered
$400 worth of drug, which is one atom away from glucose,
which he says "very likely" will be given to John. John asks,
"Will it destroy the tumor?" Jacobs says, "Yes, John, it
will."*

*I tell John he can withstand a lot and that everything's
going to be all right.*

*Chahinian and Karen Chamberlin in later: John to be put
on different IV with many more calories. Also this will help
the skin around his bedsore to heal faster.*

*This drug is the miracle if they decide to give it to him.
(Jacobs in library every night, he says, looking for reasons
not to give it to J., which might harm him.) Also, this kind
of tumor producing glucose has been seen in only thirty to
forty previous cases. "Very rare," says Jacobs.*

WEDNESDAY, DECEMBER 13, 1978

*"My greatest, deepest needs will be met by God." Wish
on a star coming home at 11:00 p.m. last night from Rodd
and Janet's in cab looking at sky on 86th Street crossway.
Star light, star bright, first star I see tonight. I wish I may,
I wish I might have the wish I wish tonight: Let John live,
let John live!*

*Sonogram results: diffuse tumorous masses attached to
intestines.*

John seems sort of low and impatient today. I feel so inad-

equate that I can't do anything for him or cheer him up. I leave him a note I wrote earlier in the day about my conviction that he has the strength and will to withstand this new drug and that everything will be all right. God will answer our prayers on this I am sure. John has the greatest determination to live for me, for his child, for his work.

. . . Tomorrow will be another miracle day, a happy, happy day. John will be given the drug, and it will work. I foresee a weekend of great thanksgiving and joy as we receive news of the tumor's destruction. I believe this miracle is possible, as John will not have it any other way. Please, God, I pray for this with every atom of my heart, soul, mind, body. I beg for this miracle.

DECEMBER 13, 1978

Dearest Bunky,

I thought about you so much last night. I am absolutely confident that your strength, courage, and determination will make this new drug work for you. I hope they don't take too long in deciding whether or not to give it to you.

I know I don't have to tell you how I long for you to be back home with me. This apartment is not home without you. I hope so much you'll be able to come home soon, healthy, happy, and strong.

Your love and thoughts of me help me every day as we approach the birth of our baby. I know I have nothing to be afraid of. I hope my deep love has the same effect on you! As I said yesterday, I know everything's going to be all right.

I love you!
Nini

THURSDAY, DECEMBER 14, 1978

Not a great day. Appointment with Dr. Uscher, who

*asks if I'm getting any rest. I guess I must look lousy. He
does an examination to determine pelvic size. Will decide
during labor and after X-ray if cesarean necessary.*

*Come back and after lunch take a nap until 3:00. I do not
visit John today but call instead. He has catheter in for new
intravenous glucose nourishment solution with many calories, which is to make him feel stronger. I talk to Dr. Jacobs
on phone, who tells me that John will be given the drug but
that it is going to take time to write up the protocol—
because he's had a variety of drugs prior to this next one.
Jacobs thinks John will receive "the agent" next week.
Christmas decorations and a tree are up on 6 North.*

*Impossible to get rings off my fingers, they are so
swollen. Feel very depressed today. Later a call—John has
been moved to 623B because they couldn't get water bed into
his room. New phone number.*

*Watch two-hour Nobel Prize documentary on this year's
winners their backgrounds, plus coverage of the cer-
emonies.*

*I wish the baby were here. I really don't look forward to
being in my eighth-floor Harkness room all by myself with
no visits from Bunky. I guess this was a day to feel sorry for
myself. Tomorrow will be better, and I will be happier.*

FRIDAY, DECEMBER 15, 1978

*John much better today when I arrive at 3:15. Very alert
and asking me about condition of house, should we get Jones
to check on it, had Rodd and Janet been staying there, how
much money did we have, that I should pay Wiedel and
Lisio before December 31, life insurance at KDW still effec-
tive in '79 even if he doesn't work, for me to get list back
from Suzanne of those people to send firm announcements
of his partnership to, that I should get extra bunches of announcements for his father and for him.*

John tells me new drug to be given to him when his white count is better (possibly by Tuesday) and that it will be for four or five days as they increase dosage. Intravenous now has high-calorie stuff going through. Also is on vitamins and, Esther tells me, a painkiller. Legs and feet a bit swelled. Stomach seems larger. John asks me if it feels soft.

He wants to listen to Pavarotti tape. Asks to be alone after I explain how the tape recorder works. It is so hard for him to press the buttons down. Asks that I buy a lightweight portable radio ("Get me the best, Nini") with earplug attachment and bring it to him tomorrow along with a copy of Sports Illustrated!

When I return from group, I help him eat a few mouthfuls of dinner. He at least drinks a pint of milk. I swear his hair is growing back.

SATURDAY, DECEMBER 16, 1978

Not a good day for John—so weak, face so gray and sunken. I bring up radio that I bought across the street. He seems very happy with it and with the earphone attachment. He tells me though to go to the waiting room for a half hour and then come back. I go in, and there are Esther and Vincent and Mom. It is so warm in there, and I am so tired. I go back and say goodbye and goodnight to John. I think John unhappy I am leaving but tells me to take care of myself. He calls me as I get to the door. "Nini, do me a favor." I walk back. The blue plastic urinal is on the table-tray across his bed. He asks me how much urine is in it—one thing they've been worried about is that John is not producing enough urine every day, so for the past week it has been monitored and recorded daily. I look and tell him 50cc. John asks me to dump it in the toilet and write down 250cc on the record sheet. I look at him. "It's okay. Just do it, Nini." I write the 250cc down with the time, and when I return with the washed-out urinal, John is lying on his side, his arm crooked up under his head, the bare forearm so thin, thin even above the elbow, no bigger than my wrist, and then hidden under the cap sleeve of the hospital gown. There is nothing so sad as a man's forearm and elbow exposed in a hospital gown. He is so weak, so fragile. He looks up at me, and I lean over and say, "I'll see you tomorrow. I love you," and then give him a kiss. And as I straighten up, his lips purse together as if there are ashes or lemons in his mouth. I pat his hand. Again he says, "Take care of yourself, Little One. Get some rest, you look tired. I'll see you tomorrow, beautiful." I nod my head and say goodbye. I wave as I make my way out of the room, getting past the two visitors Mr. Valdez has sitting at the end of his bed.

I come home with Mom, who then goes to the King Tut exhibit with Dad. I listen to Aida on the radio, maybe John is still listening to it on the new radio, and go out to the kitchen to make rum balls. The fruit cakes and now these rum balls. I have to continue our Christmas traditions even though John's not here. I am so depressed. I must not have such a hopeless feeling. I had hoped that the high-caloric intravenous would show some immediate benefit to John, but instead he is so weak.

"Faith is believing in things when common sense tells you not to." "The lovely intangibles are the only things worthwhile in life." From Miracle on 34th Street movie I am watching right now this evening. Had never seen it, but it's making me feel a little better, a little happier, a little more happier.

Please God, let John live. Even if he has to live in a hospital bed and a wheelchair here, even if we have to have nurses here every day. John's son or daughter must have the privilege of knowing him as a father. He will be able to teach him/ her even from a hospital bed. Please, God, let me too have more time with him. I want to keep on being his wife—not

*his widow. Grant this miracle please during the Christmas
season. Let me and John "be great in '78 and fine in '79!"*

SUNDAY, DECEMBER 17, 1978

*All I can repeat to myself are Emily Dickinson's words,
"After great [loss? pain? sadness?] a formal feeling comes."
A "formal feeling" that insists I be dignified, crushed in-
side, but dignified.*

*Dr. Cheung at Mt. Sinai called at 7:00 a.m. to say John
had just died. He calls back a few minutes later to read
autopsy and medical research permission papers to me over
the phone. Conversation and my verbal permission were
tape-recorded and witnessed by Miss Weeks, the operator. I
call John's parents. I tell Dad, who comes on after I tell
Uncle Jack to get him. The inevitable that we all hid from
has happened. Dad replies in yeses and nos. The silences are
awesome. There are no words that he or I can say. The tears
come when I hang up. It is real.*

*Call Msgr. Wilders at St. Thomas More, who directs me
to Mr. Rooney at Frank E. Campbell. I go there with Mom,
and he is so nice. Tells me to go to Walter B. Cooke (he
drives us there), as it will be $500 less there.*

*Then go see Msgr. Wilders. Memorial Service will be
10:00 a.m. Wednesday, December 20. Msgr. Wilders
blessed the baby as I left his office and told me that God
would give me the strength to go on.*

*Talk to Dr. Uscher, Dr. Chahinian, Dr. Lisio. Comfort-
ing calls.*

Write obituary notice and call The New York Times. *I
ask my father, "Does it sound all right?"*

*Sheryl Rubinstein comes in and stays for lunch of sand-
wiches from the deli. Dr. Uscher calls later and says he'll be
in the city and would like to stop by, which he does. We talk
about the Opera Club and that his parents and parents-in-*

law had boxes there at the Met. Then David and Carolyn
Clark stop by with Gregory asleep in the carriage.

I keep thinking the worst thing is that I'll never have
another conversation with John. I could always tell him my
problems, worries, phobias, angers, and he'd always listen.
I'll never hear him call my name again. "Oh, Nini! Where's
the Little One? How's old Short and Round? Don't ever
leave me, Nini. Do you love me, Nini?"

The wind and God are raging a tempest outside—the
wind roars. I don't think God wanted John as a permanent
resident with him so early in his life, and perhaps this wild
wind is how He is showing His anger.

But God is going to help me through these days and
through the even rougher ones months and years ahead.
Little Kate or John will give me so much to think about and
to do. What a precious gift my darling Bunky has left me.

MONDAY, DECEMBER 18, 1978
12:30 A.M.

Dear Lizzie,

A night of not being able to sleep, so I am writing to you.
I know your arms and love are around me as I tell you that
John died yesterday morning at 7:00 a.m. He was so brave
and uncomplaining to the end. And God granted to me my
prayer that his mind be alert and his body in little pain until
the end. For this I am truly grateful. We even listened to a
little bit of the Metropolitan Opera broadcast of Aida on
Saturday afternoon in his room in Mt. Sinai.

Perhaps only you and my mother know how deeply in
love I was with John and how my life and survival seemed so
connected to his need of me. I will soon have our baby and
feel somehow that such living proof of John's love, and God
too, will give me the strength to live without him.

It has been a living nightmare, and I just pray that no one

will ever have to go through what John and I have been through. It all still seems so terribly cruel.

I receive comfort though from realizing how many people admired John and thought he was one of the finest of young men. I know you and Woody, as briefly as you knew him, felt that way about him. John seemed to sparkle that evening at Susie Weist's, and I'm so glad you saw him like that.

I know your prayers are with me. Please pray that this baby be healthy and normal. I guess I won't believe it until I see it; this baby must be physically and mentally perfect. I quake with fear that something might be wrong.

I think of you, Lizzie, taking confident and healthy strolls as you regain your own strength. Please take a walk in your neighborhood for me with your head held high and know what an important, dear friend you are to me.

Take care, and all my love to you and Woody.

Nancy

CHAPTER EIGHT

I couldn't say goodbye to John, see him after he died, because to have gone into Mt. Sinai to see him would have meant he was dead in spirit as well as in flesh. No, his alive face is what I had to remember; not a dead, vacant face not knowing who I was. It would have been one thing perhaps, and only perhaps, if he'd died while I was visiting and in the room, but the fact that he died without me, and without my witnessing the slow natural passage of life to death, which might have taken some of the awfulness and foreignness out of it, made it impossible for me, for my mind, for my completing my pregnancy, to go to look at him, dead. I needed his alive spirit too much to help me through the days ahead, his memorial service, the birth of our child. I had to keep some part of him, and it had to be his spirit, his sense of life and joy, alive for myself. It was a matter of survival.

I was in shock. After I wrote Lizzie, I listened to the rain and sat in the dark night on my bed with Leo on my lap. I didn't sleep. At five-thirty I decided to take a shower and wash my hair, why, I don't know, but then I thought that as the service was going to be in St. Thomas More, it would be smart to go there once and sit there so that on Wednesday it wouldn't seem so strange. I was glad the service could be in a neighborhood family church that I'd walked by since childhood and not the grand, enormous church of John's and my wedding on 66th and Lexington. I don't think I would have been able to stand that. The picture taken of John and me beaming and smiling to the guests as we passed their pews on our way out after the ceremony was too vivid. That healthy young man beside me. No, I could not have sat in that same church.

I quietly left the apartment a little before seven, my mother asleep. Twenty-four hours ago, I was thinking, John was dying. I walked to 89th Street and the church. It was a cold Monday morning, and when I entered the church I saw that the seven-o'clock mass had just begun. There were older women and a few older men scattered in the pews. One young woman there with her little daughter. I wondered why. Who were they praying for? I sat and stared up at the stained-glass window above the altar. Jesus, Mary, little lambs, some doves. The circle showing Mary with the infant Jesus. Maybe that will help on Wednesday, I thought, I'll look at that, a mother holding a child. I didn't know what to pray for as I sat there. It was very hard to believe there was a God. I hoped John was all right wherever he was. Was he crossing the River Styx? I still needed him. I prayed to God, though, for the safety of John's and my baby. I told myself, as John would have told me, that everything was going to be all right. "Just don't worry about it, Nini."

I left and went into the deli on the corner and got a cup of coffee to go. It was warm in my gloved hands as I walked the two blocks to the 90th Street entrance of the park. I walked up the steps to the reservoir, and took off the plastic lid, and watched the steam of the coffee swirl in the wind. I walked across the narrow running track and looked through the diamond shaped openings of the metal chain-link fence out to the water and to the buildings on Central Park West, the sun beginning to shine on them. I saw and heard seagulls flying over the reservoir, and they made me cry. Why wouldn't I ever see John running into the water, running up and down the beach, lumbering out of the ocean, hearing him say, "Come on in, Nini, the water's glorious"? What about our walks on the beach that last summer, how Bunky would never wear shoes, so his feet would burn on the hot sand, deck, and parking lot? I stood there and couldn't believe he was gone. I followed with my eyes the flight of the seagulls and, hearing footsteps, stepped back next to the stone railing at the top of the steps to let a runner pass. Below me was the bridle path where John and I ran together in the mornings before work. I could almost pretend I saw him there, still running backward, laughing and holding his arms high up in the air, saying, as I followed him, "Hey, you're a good runner, Little One, you're doing fine." Another runner climbed the steps to get to the running track—could have been any young NYC lawyer type—he looked at me as I tried to stop crying, covering my face with a Kleenex. I wiped my eyes and nose as if I had a cold, a terrible runny nose, but it probably didn't fool him. I smiled at him, and he looked relieved and started his run. It was time to go. I couldn't let anyone else see me crying.

I tossed the empty coffee container into the trash basket, and with my hands deep in my pockets and my eyes on the ground, I started walking home. I went over to Madison Avenue, and before me I saw one of my favorite Nightingale girls walking toward me on her way to school; I'd forgotten it was a Monday, a school day. What was I going to say? She saw me and she looked as if she felt as awkward as I did. "Hi, Jennifer."

"Hi, Mrs. Rossi."

"I've just been walking in the park. My husband died yesterday."

"Yes, I know," said Jennifer. "I heard about it yesterday at the pageant." I'd forgotten. Nightingale's biannual Christmas pageant had been yesterday. I looked at her. She was only fourteen and I was twenty-nine, and all I could do was bite my lip while her eyes looked sad and scared. God, I didn't want to scare her. I felt like an alien, a freak, and I could tell she felt sorry for me. I think I patted her on the shoulder, and I think she patted me on the shoulder, too. We both nodded our heads, and as I felt the tears about to come again, I gave a wave with my fingers and said, "I'll see you, Jennifer," and continued walking. Oh, dear, I worried she would never forget this, that she saw black-coated Mrs. Rossi walking on Madison Avenue the morning after her husband died. Nothing made any sense. How would my life go on? I wondered. How would I be able to handle other people's pity? The safest way seemed to be to become the stoic widow, cool, withdrawn, avoiding at any cost having others hug me or tell me they understood.

I got back to the apartment. Notes and flowers had begun to arrive. Esther and Vincent and Aunt Linuccia arrived with John's things from the hospital in a regular brown paper bag that hospitals use. Aching, wrenching time. The women all cried. Mr. Rossi tried to settle us, to soothe us. He tried so hard as Esther and I held each other, she patting my head as John would have, and the two of us sobbing, "He was too young!" Underneath the unbearable grief was rage. We had all been fooled into believing that a good, kind, honest life would be rewarded. John's death rocked us to cynicism. I asked Esther if she wanted any of John's things, clothes or anything. No, she wouldn't be able to bear it. They left to drive back to Croton.

I was like a zombie all afternoon. After dinner with my parents, my mother and I took a walk in the icy, clear night air up to 90th Street and back. On Fifth Avenue she mentioned remembering having seen Robert Kennedy and Jackie Kennedy walking along Fifth, past the Guggenheim Museum, one evening maybe six months after JFK had been assassinated, both in earnest conversation as they walked. My mother's meaning from that was that one must take walks, get outside. My instant understanding of her story, having once waited for the Wall Street Express bus across the street from her apartment and seeing an elderly Mr. Onassis walking his dog, was that no one—not the media, no one—should have been allowed to judge her, her remarriage, her always chronicled extravagance, none of it, because no one had lived through what she had. Already I could tell others were going to be giving me advice—get out, see friends, don't be alone— and thinking of her, her aloof, quiet dignity, gave me the courage to be the woman I wanted to be at John's service.

As we walked outside, the cold air blowing over us, I was hoping that the New Jersey wind from the west, which always passes over the city, maybe had atoms of John in it. He had been cremated in New Jersey that day.

Again without much sleep I awakened early the day

of the service. How many pregnant women have had "widow's weeds"? Black was not a color that would have been in my maternity wardrobe. I chose the last thing John saw me in. A gray-blue paisley wool dress. I hated it as I put it on. I'd rather have worn red, white, anything, but this would have to do. As we walked to the church, Tony Schlesinger gave me an envelope. A letter from him, a beautifully worded reminiscence of the past summer and his tennis playing and Dickens reading with John. I held it throughout the service; it, too, gave me strength.

The service was not as bad as I had thought it was going to be, actually very positive, comforting and uplifting. A celebration, Msgr. Wilders called it. Heaven is not full of angels playing harps in Elysian Fields, but a oneness with God. A place where there is no suffering or death. I began to cry when the singer started "Amazing Grace," John's favorite hymn; "Panis Angelicus" during the time people came up for Communion. Gave me a chance to look around the church. It was packed; people standing in the back. I gripped my brother's hand during the rest of the service, my older brother by eight years, the one who in my childhood always looked out for me. I needed him now. It ended. It appeared I was to be the first to leave. There's protocol, just as at a wedding. I gave my coat to my brother to hold, odd thing to do, and even odder, I followed the motioning hands that were telling me to get up and leave, and walk out alone. I think my brother wanted to catch up with me, to hold my arm, but I was determined to leave alone. Eight and a half months pregnant, and I wanted everyone to see: that I was pregnant and alone. When I got to the alcove of the church entrance, where I guessed I was to stand to "receive condolences," I saw Esther and Vincent walk toward me arm in arm, Esther crumpling like a ball of squeezed, wet Kleenex; Vincent, her husband, supporting her frail, tiny mass. Somehow, by whom I don't know, we were lined up near the door. All the girls it seemed who knew me at Nightingale were there, the headmistress, the teachers. I didn't realize until then how much it meant to me to see that packed church begin to file out and stand waiting to say a few words to me and our families. All, it seemed, of Kelley Drye, all our Bayberries friends, Raymond the doorman, the superintendent of the building, the members of the building's board of directors, the Community Service Society board members that John and David worked with, John's secretary, childhood friends of John's and mine, even some of the doctors.

Afterward there was a brief gathering in the apartment. Sherry and coffee and tea and little breakfast pastries. How odd to see these dainty treats on trays that had known other foods in happier dinner-party-giving days. Trays that John would have carried. After standing and talking for a while I felt I had to sit down. I apologized to the fellow I was talking to, one of John's friends from the office, and told him I was getting tired—"No, please, keep talking, Alvin, you're making me laugh, I just have to sit down." He said, "It's about time." These were our families and best friends. No one was going to say anything dumb. Yet I went to bed that night thinking that the only thing I didn't understand was the notion that John had now found peace, as he was the only person I'd ever known who found peace in living.

The next morning I still had the queer notion on and off all day that John wasn't really gone, that he would return. I was glad Mr. Foote from the 6 North desk told me he was there when John died, as it made it seem more real. Bill and Sheryl called and told me how dignified I was during and after the service. That meant a lot, as I knew John would have said, "Nini, you did good." He would have been proud of me. I wondered, though, would I ever be "the queen of my heart, the light of my life, goddess of the east wind and west" to anyone again? I loved being married. It's the sharing I was going to miss so much.

Before the Rossis left with John's ashes for Utica, John's brother, Vincent, and his sister Tisha came in to help me go through John's clothes. My mother said to me recently, "I had to get those clothes out of there; I was afraid you were going to stand and stare into that open closet with all his clothes forever." Oddly, Vincent, Tisha and I laughed over some memories his clothes brought back. We were all in shock. Everything was packed to be picked up by Cancer Care except items Vincent and Tisha wanted and John's old tennis hat, which I kept. His watch, the formal shirt studs from Tiffany's, his grandfather's gold cufflinks from our opera days and his fountain pen were packed in his jewelry box for his son or daughter. His books were still on the bookshelves throughout the house. The main impression though was how little a man owns. His clothes, his books, a watch. Not much. It is for others that men buy and give things. I could not bear it when I packed his jogging suit and his running shoes into one of the boxes. I was glad though never to have to see again those huge size-44-waist gray flannel pants. But then his underwear and sock drawers. It was awful. It all still smelled of him. And I didn't want it to be taken from me so soon, but I said nothing.

Every year, year after year, the week after John's death is Christmas Eve and the week after that is New Year's Eve: 17th, 24th, 31st. It was impossible to believe that Christmas Eve would come so soon, and that night I wished I could believe in the real Christmas story and its joyful tidings, but I couldn't. My sorrow seemed so huge. I pictured John alone and cold in the Utica ground. I was too near giving birth to be allowed to go to Utica for the funeral service there and to the family plot in the cemetery. All through this siege I kept thinking, It should be me—I'm the one for whom living is so difficult and such a fearful chore most of the time. I thought that perhaps I should be grateful that he was not spending Christmas Eve on 6 North, but it didn't help. My father, thinking it would cheer me up, had me open a gift from him. A new camera. I burst into tears. That's what *I* was going to give John before any of this started, a camera for him to take pictures of our baby. It was not my father's fault, but it hit me the wrong way. The last thing I wanted was a camera. I didn't want anything. It even seemed sick to think of Christmas presents.

However, I was determined to be cheerful for my nieces on Christmas Day. They were only little girls, nine and five; I could not ruin their day. My brother, Sandy, and his girlfriend, Doris, did everything in their power to give the girls, me, my parents a candlelit perfect-tree Christmas in their apartment on 86th Street. We ignored the fact that, except for Sandy and Doris buying presents at the last minute for all of us, the rest of us had not bought anything except gifts for the girls. Yesterday's awful gift of the camera was forgotten. I was glad when the day was over. I spoke to the Rossis in Utica. We were all numb. None of it made any sense except to ourselves. Wishes of Merry Christmas were so absurd they weren't said. It was a grim day, and I yearned for Christmas the next year when I would have a child to think about.

The mail the next day continued to bring piles of sympathy letters. One packet in the middle, in a brown paper envelope, was John's death certificates. I looked at them and couldn't believe they were talking about him. I had another childbirth session with the wife of a law-school friend of John's, who taught Lamaze courses in Westchester. When discussing breast-feeding, I told her that if it was too painful for me, I would stop, as "I feel I've been through enough this year, that this is not the time for me to feel I have to prove something." I didn't think she understood, she asked that I call her anytime if I thought I'd like to give up, that maybe she could help me. We talked later about John, about asbestos, mesothelioma. It brought it all back to me. I sat in the living room with Mom, trying to read *Gourmet* and *Bon Appétit*, hoping to get my mind off John so that I wouldn't cry. However, quietly I picked up Leo and went back into the bedroom and cried softly but so hard. I kept repeating, "It's not fair. I want my Bunky, I want my Uncle Buckle."

Mom would not leave me alone. I kept trying to explain that I wanted to be by myself that night. Leo, incredibly, must have understood how sad I was, as he sat on my lap or right next to me constantly. Mom had some understanding that I wanted my house back to myself again. I was tired of the fact that she only liked certain kinds of music. It was like having a guest. I had to realize how hard she was trying to do and say the right thing, that it was difficult for her, too, to be living there. I felt resentful that she kept intruding, though. As John used to say, "Granny talks too much." Everything seemed to be *"we"* had to get such and such for the baby. When the baby was there, *"we'll . . ."* But there was only one person who made up a *"we"* with me, and he was gone.

I was so depressed that 1978 was ending so soon. At least John had been a living part of 1978. He had no part in 1979. And he would have no part in all the years that were ahead for me. I was having such a hard time accepting that, that one day the pictures of him would look dated, that one day I would say to myself, "John's been dead twenty years!" Why did this tragedy have to happen to us? That question made me cry again.

I got depressed, too, thinking that the years I had with him were the only happiness I would know, that maybe others who said the reverse were wrong, that happiness and closeness with another would never come again.

I listened to the Philadelphia Orchestra under Eugene Ormandy play Shubert's Ninth Symphony. I realized that John must have listened to a WQXR program called *Woody's Children* at seven in the evening and then the Philadelphia concert later, two weeks ago tonight. It was hard to believe that the next day he would have been dead two weeks—in a way it seemed such a short time, though right then it seemed like forever. The memory of the good, healthy, alive times was so far away, and yet came upon me vividly, unexpectedly.

I was trying to concentrate on reading *The Snow Leopard* by Peter Matthiessen, thinking it would help me. Weeks before I had read in the introduction that his wife had "died of cancer, in the winter." I gathered it had been five or six years before. I wondered how he had survived. I thought I had heard that he had married again.

That day my Lamaze teacher asked me if I'd had an amniocentesis test and knew whether the baby was a boy or a girl. I said no and said I thought it better that John hadn't known either. She then said something to the effect that John knew then, even if I still didn't. For some reason, that remark offended me. How could John know whether it was a boy or girl? John was dead! I couldn't believe that he now "knew" things. I guess I could vaguely believe that he was sort of looking over me and still wanted the best for me and still wanted me to be strong and brave. But that was such a vague feeling and a feeling I could conjure up only when I felt weak or scared and I repeated his orders to be a "good girl, Nini" or to be "great in '78 and fine in '79." At those times I felt he was still talking to me, but I realized that it was only because I remembered his voice and words on similar occasions so vividly. I guess I couldn't believe that John was talking to me or "knew" what was going on in my life. And yet I could see my future behavior and living of life as a kind of tribute to him and his positive philosophy. Somehow my copying his strong and generous qualities seemed a good thing to try to do, and not crazy. I truly believed he came into my life to teach me a few things. And as my tribute to him I thought I had learned them well enough so as to make them a part of my personality. I was then sure, too, that the baby would teach me even more about him and remind me daily of John's smile, fun, laugh. *Why* did John have to say so often, from the night I first met him in Manhasset, "When you get to be my age, every day is a gift"? It was a joke then, with me and others replying, "Sure, John, you're so old!" But it wasn't funny now.

A few days later I took a walk in the rain to the park and then sat in St. Thomas More. At least it was quiet there, no phone calls, no sympathy letters, and nobody talked to me. My feet and fingers were so swollen. I was really looking forward to seeing whether the baby would be a girl or a boy *and* to getting rid of that huge stomach and the swelling in my hands and feet.

This day was better than the one before, when I cried most of the day. Rodd and Janet stopped by in the afternoon with a beautiful caftan/robe as a Christmas present from them and Diane. Things were better with Mom, too. Before I had been jealous of pregnant women; now I was jealous of husbands and wives. I should be grateful for what I have when I have it. I guess.

I was all packed for the hospital. Had to get a few more things the next day, like a small bottle of shampoo, but other than that I was all set.

I got a call from David and Teri Barry—Kelley Drye friends—that night, which was nice, but Teri said, when praising what a joy babies are, "We go to bed each night so happy with the day we've had with her." I would be going to bed alone with nobody to share the fun or exasperation with. Except Leo the cat. If John couldn't return, I wished someone like him would come into my life and want me and love me. I was so lonely without John. I could hear him saying, "Now don't worry, Nini, be a good girl. Remember, life by the yard is hard; life by the inch is a cinch. You've just got to have more confidence in yourself, Nini! You get more beautiful every day, Nini."

I called John's father to tell him about Workmen's Compensation claims. I would mail them to him. He sounded well and strong. Later that evening I called Vincent Jr. and had a good chat. I couldn't sleep for some reason that night, even though I had to be at Dr. Uscher's at nine in the morning. I hoped Dr. Uscher would say that the baby would be on time! I couldn't wait for a more regular, normal life to begin, with me independent and head of my own house.

JANUARY 3, 1979

Dear Lizzie,

After I read your first letter after John died, I kept saying to myself that your understanding of what John and I had been through was so complete it was as if you were here and not in London. We both tried so hard to be the persons we'd each married, showing still the same qualities that made us love each other so much, right to the end. The extent of John's huge effort in this regard was made clear to me only last week with the autopsy report: the tumor had grown right through his diaphragm and was starting to grow into his right lung—in fact, there was no organ in the trunk of his body that was not affected. The pain he must have been in that he never let on about, his determination to protect his "Little One" from the hideous agony he was going through, was so typically him. He never raged against this unfunny roll of the dice or complained.

I felt I had truly not given him much in the way of understanding or comfort, but I see that just being myself, still gently teasing him, as I was the only one who could look beyond the physical and see a John who in spite of his illness hadn't changed very much at all, was what he appreciated most. That is why I was so moved by your saying that I let him die without guilt. You are the only one who has seen that.

I was running around last week paying doctor bills before the end of '78 and was able to talk to John's surgeon at Presbyterian. I told him I'd felt bad that John had never wanted to discuss his dying with me or anyone else, and the surgeon, who does just about all of the exploratory operations for tumors there, said it is the very rare patient who does want to talk about his death, that everyone "wants to leave quietly." That certainly was John. I then thanked the doctor for his gentle yet honest manner in breaking the results of the operation to me while John was still in the recovery room. It is amazing that even now I remember every word he said. He told me, as John's other doctors have told me, that breaking news like that gets harder, not easier, no matter how many times one has done it, especially when a young person is involved. I've since learned that doctors' lounges are equipped with boxes of Kleenex for their own crying either before or after telling a patient's family hopeless findings.

Now receiving your Christmas Eve letter today shows again how close you are in understanding my current emotional barometer. Unfortunately, you're right, it does get worse as the days go by, not better. The picture of the ill John recedes, and I start thinking of the boundless, healthy John who, it seems to me, should be turning the key in the lock and racing in here. That's when I've got to remind myself of what torture he was in, because if I don't, I can't understand at all why he isn't here. Thoughts of what the baby's birth certificate will say, of being on that maternity floor with no husband to visit me, are so terrible and hurt so much that they literally, it seems, throw me against a wall. I then think, "This has never happened to anyone." Of course, that isn't true. . . .

One thing that does keep me from going off the deep end is the cancer therapy group I'd been going to while John was ill and continue to go to now. At first after John died I wasn't sure if I wanted to go back, as I was the first in the group to have the husband or wife die, that I might be too depressing for them, and that I'd be terribly jealous of them and their still-living spouses. But as it turns out, and with the encouragement of the doctor and social worker who run it that I must not stop going, and even though it hurts terribly to go there and talk every week, I know if I do stop I will lose my chance at recovery, at understanding, and at the possibility of relearning how to accept joy and happiness into my life. I am determined in a way to make a completely new start with my life, to leave behind old fears and feelings of incompetence. One of the first actual demonstrations of this is going to be getting my driver's license and buying a car. I never thought I was going to be able to drive on the Long Island Expressway, but I see that fear as so petty now.

Also, I've managed to get myself to one Christmas-season party and have been able to see friends for lunch, etc., without its bothering me too much, although I can't tell you what a tremendous effort it takes, for, again, you are right, nobody wants to see anyone but the cheerful, optimistic Nancy, because they don't know how to react should I be sad. It is a burden, as you said, but one that is actually a lot easier than my having to put up with their inarticulateness. It's been very hard to accept, with good grace and not want-

ing to smack the person who says it, expressions of "I un-
derstand" from those who so obviously never could. . . .

The only sense I get of John's "presence" is really just
happy memories—memories of his words of encouragement
to me in the past and the happiness I feel walking around his
adored running track in the park and my remembering how
proud he was of me with my own running progress. But to
actually think he's there is ridiculous. I also can be hit sud-
denly with thinking how John would either have loved a
particular day, meal, or some such that I am now enjoying
or how he would have hated it. So the memory of his reac-
tions to things, which I knew so well, also keeps him
around, but only in my mind, and that to me is all there is
to "life after death"—just people's memories of you alive in
their minds. . . .

Always there are going to be pieces of music, watching
Jimmy Connors play tennis, a foggy morning in Bridge-
hampton when we'd see rabbits and pheasants, that are
going to make me painfully aware of his no longer being
here, and I wouldn't want it any other way, but to count
on these moments as a future way of life seems sick to me
and definitely not something John would approve of!

Even though I write in a diary every night, I find these
rambling letters that I can write to you such good therapy
for me. I hope you don't mind that I find it so easy to "talk"
to you on paper. It is so obvious to me that you understand
that I may take advantage of your patient listening. I'm
sure you'd rather hear news of NYC and of funny stories in
the Times! Sharing my grief with you seems unfair to you,
but I've wanted you so much to understand that your life
with Woody is more precious and more important than ever
getting pregnant. Please don't feel left out of the human
race, as I used to feel when month after month went by,
because a husband is much more important. There can be no
substitute for sharing a married life with another. Somehow

if what I've been through helps you to accept a life with Woody as a full life and a happy, worthwhile life, then certainly I take that as a bit of happiness and good out of this avalanche of sadness. . . .

I hope my next letter has news of the baby. I'm getting the feeling the baby's planning to skip winter and instead arrive on Memorial Day!

All my love,
Nancy

It got worse and worse. I cried and cried. And Dr. Uscher said the baby was going to be two weeks late! I had a terrible fight with my mother one night. Our living together in my apartment, she to watch over me, had exploded. She went back to live in her own apartment. I needed peace. I needed my home back, John's and my home back. I had to refind John here alone, to adjust alone. I had to be able to cry without her rushing in. I got the most angry when she gave me the impression I was not capable.

By the baby's due date I had the flu—sore throat and cold. My feet and fingers were swollen, and Dr. Uscher told me to stay off my feet for at least five hours a day. I still felt there must have been some mistake, that the sick John was dead but that the healthy, breezy John would still come back into my life someday. What a road to torture. I had to get over that feeling; it would produce nothing, just a running away from deadening grief before I could live again. Anne Morrow Lindbergh's preface to the year 1932 in her diaries, really an essay on grief, on the different stages of mourning—numbness, almost a false courage and stoicism, remorse and self-pity, then vulnerability that will lead to eventual rebirth, in other words learning how to love and be loved again—was the only written word that helped. The Bible was remote. Even the Psalms.

I forced myself to watch John McEnroe beat Arthur Ashe in the final of a tennis tournament on television. How happy everyone at Bayberries had been the year that Ashe beat Connors at Wimbledon, but this day I was happy McEnroe beat Ashe, I guess because of how similar McEnroe's tennis is to John's. And even as I missed John so terribly, watching the match reminded me of so many happy Sundays in the past when John would be watching "the tennis," as he called it, and I would be making dinner and periodically would come in to get the score—those memories made me happy and made me think the happiness in my life was not over. But the next moment I was in tears again, still not understanding that hideous asbestos. I tried to find the healthy John by going through old photographs, so few of them, so few of us together, and our wedding album. Was that asbestos sitting there in his body the day of our wedding, just waiting to start its rampage? The answer was yes.

A letter from Esther had arrived that day. She understood my loss of John. I wrote her back right away. I thought I understood her and Vincent's loss of John better today myself, as their dream of the future had been in John, their firstborn. Our clawing animosity was over. We were friends. And we discovered in future years, after others were tired and uninterested in our memories of John, that she and I could talk openly about John only to each other, that neither of us tired of remembering him.

A month after John's death I began to have some crampy pains. I tried to decide if they were labor pains, and when they stopped after three hours I decided they were not. And then a week later after fixing myself a piece of chicken for dinner the cramps started again. Nothing regular, but the baby was moving around a lot. I was not going to bother anyone yet. I went back to the bookcases outside the baby's room and tried to find the author of "thy beauty is to me like those Nicean barks of yore," which John used to say about me, and went through his collection of poetry books. I came across Tennyson's "Lady of Shalott" and remembered that John could recite the entire poem. What a memory he had. I missed him so much, and there seemed to be less and less of him near me there in the apartment. He had gotten so far away so fast that it was hard to remember him living there. It was awful, but I could hear him say, "Go to sleep, Nini. Get some rest, Nini. Nighty-night, Nini." I even had my first dream of him that night; he was asking me where breakfast was.

At three in the morning I woke up with what had to be labor pains, and I got out a yellow legal pad from John's old office files and started timing them until five o'clock, when they came every four minutes. The apartment was still and quiet; I went to the dining room to watch the rain, blasts of rain were being blown by the wind up Madison Avenue under the street lights. I turned on the radio. It was five-thirty. Figured I'd better call Dr. Uscher. The phone wasn't working. I couldn't get a dial tone. I kept pressing "O" for Operator—nothing. I called down to the lobby on the house phone and asked the night doorman if there was a phone I could use in the basement. No, there wasn't any phone, he said. That surprised me, as I could have sworn there was one in a room off the lobby leading to the fire stairs. There was nothing to be done. I packed my suitcase, got dressed and walked in the rain to my mother's apartment. What a sight I must have been: a not-even-five foot tall swollen pregnant woman, holding an umbrella, a suitcase and a handbag, walking in the rain before dawn. I didn't see anybody else on the streets.

The doorman at my mother's building rang her apart-

ment. No answer. I told him she probably had the humidi-
fier on and couldn't hear his buzzing, so he let me go on
up. I rang and rang the doorbell and knocked too—she
couldn't hear that either. Jesus Christ. I went back downstairs and called her on the telephone in the lobby. Her
phone rang in her bedroom and she answered. I could
hardly talk, the story was so bizarre and there was so
much to explain, but I told her my phone was out and
could I call Dr. Uscher from her apartment? It didn't even
occur to me to call him from her lobby phone or from the
pay phone on the corner. For one who was determined to
have this baby all by herself, it turned out I needed my
mother after all.

Dr. Uscher told me to go to the hospital. He would meet
me there. Even though he was off duty that weekend, he
had reassured me earlier that no one but he was going to
deliver this special baby. Next I phoned for a taxi to take
us to Columbia-Presbyterian. It was still raining very hard,
and there were no cabs on the street.

The doorman called up that the cab was there, and in
the six-a.m. dark we sped up the West Side Highway. The
young driver didn't know how to get to 168th Street and
the hospital. I had to give him directions.

On the labor floor nothing much had changed from the
time I had been there in 1975. The fetal monitor was
strapped on, and dumbly I sat in the bed staring at the
monitor, as if it were a television screen, with my mother
sitting in a chair next to it. At last I was going to see the
baby; I tried not to think about John. The contractions
were starting to hurt, and I was glad I was going to have a
cesarean.

When Dr. Uscher arrived, he wheeled me down to the
X-ray room, just to make sure that the baby's head was in
fact too big to get through "your teeny pelvis." It was, and

we headed back upstairs, me to be prepped for the operation, he to change out of his Levi's.

The delivery room had rows of windows on two sides,
looking south over Manhattan and west over the river.
This was a first, an operating room with windows and not
surrounded by green tile. It was now eleven o'clock and
the sun was shining. The residents draped the familiar
green cloth on a metal holder over my chest to form a curtain. Dr. Uscher came in quite relaxed, and he agreed with
the two anesthesiologists that because of my sore throat
and cold, I should have a spinal anesthetic instead of the
general, which uses a tube inserted down one's throat.
They asked me to sit up and bend over, and the needle
was carefully positioned at the base of my spine and then
inserted. I lay back down and waited for whatever was
supposed to happen, and all of a sudden I got scared and
panicked. I sat back up and they asked what was wrong. I
said nothing, I was just a little scared. They asked me to
please lie down again, and Dr. Uscher started talking
about how he was going to have to bail water out of his
basement when he got back home. Said the driveway was
a lake with all the rain the night before and early that
morning.

The two anesthesiologists started talking about the spinal; I'd be numb from the waist down. Did I feel it yet?
Yes. They pricked me in a few places; I could feel nothing.
It was weird. The woman anesthesiologist agreed but said
the weirdest sensation she had ever had was when she
had had a spinal that numbed her from the neck down:
"It's very peculiar not to be able to feel your own breathing!" I relaxed. At least I could still feel my chest rise and
fall with each breath. The other anesthesiologist was a
British man about my age. He was here on a fellowship he
told me. He and the woman were chatting above my head,

and my eyes went from one to the other to follow the conversation. Dr. Uscher was farther down the table telling his residents what to do. "Wait till you see the incision I did for her ectopic. Now look, see, great work, huh?" He and the residents and the nurses were laughing. "Okay," he said, "we're ready to go."

I didn't feel anything as he discussed how he was cutting through the layers of skin, then fat. He told me I would feel a tug when he lifted the baby out. The room was still. I felt the tug, and looked at his gloved hands and arms reaching down behind the curtain, and then in a second he was bringing the baby up to my line of vision, holding the baby under the armpits, the umbilical cord still twisting down, and his voice choked—they all knew there was no husband there and why—and he practically shouted, "Oh, Nance, it's a *boy*! It's a *boy*!"

"Oh," I sighed, "it is?"

He was there right in front of me, his face all frowning and screwing up for that first big yell, and out it came. Everyone in the room murmured, "Oh, isn't it lovely—she got a boy!"

Dr. Uscher put the baby's cheek next to my face so that I could kiss him, and for a brief moment he let the baby's and my cheeks rest together, side by side. A resident cut the umbilical cord and clamped it, and the pediatric nurse and resident took him away to be weighed.

Dr. Uscher looked up. "Anybody get the time?" The big wall clock was high on the wall. "It's now eleven thirty-two," he said. "Let's say eleven thirty-one."

I kept saying softly, "It's a boy, it's a boy." I hadn't thought I was going to have a boy; I had been sure, absolutely certain, it would be a girl. It was a surprise. I had thought I couldn't dare hope for a boy, as hoping and praying had proved to be useless. But here I'd had what I, even in my most cynical moments, had continued to pray for. A boy. John Francis Rossi III was here. And instead of feeling that I was on a table surrounded by people who could not possibly understand what this meant to me, around me were a group of men and women as moved as I by the birth of John Francis Rossi III.

Dr. Uscher and the residents began to sew me back up—Dr. Uscher at one point laughing and saying, "Hey, Nancy, you really ought to take a look at this, watch us sew you up. We're doing a terrific job here. We can take down the curtain so you can see." And I laughed back, saying, "Thanks, but I'll pass." And everyone laughed— the room became a buzz of conversation. The British fellow telling me how long he'd be here, when he'd be going home; I remember that I even opened up and said how happy John would have been, and Dr. Uscher said, "He sure would have."

By noon I was in the recovery room, the only one there. Dr. Uscher had changed back to his Levi's and said, "Well, little mother, I'll see you tomorrow. Gotta go home and bail out the house. You planned this just right, too; nobody's going to miss the Super Bowl this afternoon!" And he gave me a kiss and a strong hug to express what words couldn't. There were tears in our eyes.

My mother had called my father, and they both came into the recovery room. There had been someone in there earlier that morning, but now I had the room to myself and the nurses decided to bring the baby in and let him lie next to me on the bed. I had to keep my head down and move as little as possible, as they had warned me the spinal could cause a headache after-effect, so I slowly turned my head to the wrapped bundle they had put in the crook of my arm. And I looked at the baby's huge dark-blue eyes, the dark hair on his head, and I whispered, "Hello, John. I'm your Mommy." Seven pounds, three ounces— exactly what his father had weighed at birth.

In the hospital, when I woke up in the morning, instead of thinking, "Oh, what is it, what has gone wrong?" and realizing that it was John, "Oh, yes, John is dead," I thought, "What is it, why am I happy? Oh, I have a baby!" It was wonderful to feel happy again. But the combination of grief and happiness made for very up-and-down moods. Baskets and baskets of flowers arrived. How fast my titles had changed: wife, widow, mother.

I had a wonderful day with new John. He started nursing really well that morning and had such a dear, contented look on his face while he was eating. Whenever he started to cry, I was able to quiet him so quickly. He just seemed to know I was his mother and that I loved him very much.

What a huge grin John gave me the next day. At his six-o'clock feeding he had no trouble eating and had his eyes open looking at me the whole time. He was so easy to burp, too. As crazy as this sounds, at that moment I thought he already really loved me—I could feel it. And my love for him was a kind I'd never experienced. It certainly was as strong and wonderful as my love for his daddy, but this had an added dimension of pride and gratefulness that John and I were able to produce him. It was such a miracle. I hadn't thought I would ever experience joy or happiness again, but the moment John was lifted out of my stomach, covered with some blood, but not much, and crying, with tons of oxygen filling up his lungs, making his little chest expand back and forth, I was transported. I never dreamed having my own little boy would be so wonderful.

I loved my little John so much. I was so grateful to God for having given me this happy life to take care of.

A childhood friend whom I'd known since we were both six months old, Lynda Crowley, called, and we had a wonderful talk. She was so happy for me. I spent part of the morning packing; I was so anxious for the next day to come so that I could get John home. How nice to come home from the hospital with a healthy John. Something had become a little clearer to me when Lynda told me of her college roommate, who was now going through a nasty divorce, with fights about child-support payments and visits: that although the time allowed John and me was unbearably short, it had been happy. As Lynda had said, John had died loving me. I was so glad he had felt the baby kick. I shouldn't have been saying "the baby" anymore. I meant John. How happy I was to say that!

Dr. Lazarus, the pediatrician, came in to tell me I had an absolutely perfect and healthy baby and that the breast-feeding was going just fine. He asked me if I was depressed, and I said, "No, not really." I showed Dr. Lazarus the two pictures of healthy John in the frame, saying, "You never met the healthy John." And Dr. Lazarus said, "No, when I saw him, he was very sick."

He looked at John's pictures for a long time, looked up and said, "You don't know how many hours of sleep I've lost over this. He was my age and at the same point in life I am." He said that I had been "through the wringer" and now was the time for me to be happy and enjoy things again.

The Rossis visited with Aunt Helen, even though they had vowed never to return to New York City after their son had died. Dad and Aunt Helen were fine and upbeat; Ma started off okay, happy about my being able to call her so soon after the delivery. But when Helen and Dad left the room, she and I both cried. The unfairness of John's being gone, not being able to see his son. I had tried so hard not to think about that; I hadn't wanted to be reminded of sadness now, no matter how relevant it was, I just wanted to be happy. I called Mary Ellen, John's sister, and we had a very good talk. I told her that having John III didn't make up for everything, for the cruelty of John's death, but that the baby was a greater blessing than I had imagined he would be and that he had made me happy again.

The next day I was supposed to go to a demonstration class of how to bathe a baby, but when I heard a man's voice outside in the hall, I realized that fathers would be there, too. I told the nurse I couldn't go and explained. She understood.

I worried that going home with my parents in the car, with no husband, would be unbearable, but it wasn't too bad. Lovely Miss Robinson, the nurse the Rossis had given me for two weeks, was there waiting for us in the apartment. She was wonderful, her soft West Indian voice making the house peaceful. She knew about my husband, but she didn't ask questions.

The days after John's birth on January 21 were cold, wintery. Dr. Lazarus said John could go outside in his carriage once the temperature was above 40 degrees. And ten days later it was my thirtieth birthday. Years before, during the time of the big Bayberries thirtieth-birthday celebrations, I remember being told that mine would be a huge one because I would be the last in the group to turn thirty. Never would I have imagined that I would spend this birthday as a mother and a widow, but Rodd and Janet came over after dinner with a cake, and Sandy and Doris arrived, too, making it a party. Not a Bayberries party but a very happy one. As I wrote to Lizzie that night, "Today is my thirtieth birthday, and even a month ago, no one could have told me I'd be happy today."

I was learning the lesson that the more people told me I would be able to cope just fine and told me how well I was doing, the better I was, but when others reminded me of the rough road ahead—"You have to be father and mother"—I descended. An acquaintance who had had a baby two weeks before John was born called, and I couldn't get her to stop talking: "Those last few weeks of pregnancy are so emotional—how did you deal with them all alone? You must have felt awful. Did they decide what caused John's cancer? Don't you cry all the time with postpartum depression? I cry every night." Shit. I felt like hanging up on her. My answer was that this was a happy event, and that I didn't have the inclination to cry. It was awful. How do people think they are so fascinating to others that they can get away with such tactlessness? Then the topper—"You must be a very strong person, Nancy." Yeah, you would be, too, if you'd seen the dearest person ever to come into your life disintegrate in front of you.

A few days after that I did the strangest thing, and I wasn't even thinking about it at the time. I just picked up the phone and started dialing the Kelley Drye office number, and I realized only when the operator answered, "Kelley Drye and Warren," that I was going to say, "John Rossi, please." I hung up right away. I was getting used to the physical absence of John—except that I still missed him on the other side of our bed, at his chair at the dinner table—but what I wanted to do that afternoon was to give him a call. I just felt like talking to him, to tell him about John III and how much I was enjoying him and that I was trying my best to be a good mother, that I knew it would be difficult, and that I wished he were here to teach his son how to pee in a toilet when the time came. And it was a shock to realize I couldn't even call him.

Even though it was still too cold to take John out in his carriage, I went for walks every day, and every day I ended up at the reservoir, staring out over the water, waiting for John to turn the corner with the rest of the runners. That seemed to be my "widow's walk." On Valentine's Day I was there "telling" John I was still his Valentine. I spent more and more time looking at the pictures I had of him, and each time I got that old startle of realization that he was not coming back. When I thought I was going to start to cry, I told myself to stop it, right then. I had to be strong for the baby.

I thought maybe I would feel better if I made plans to get my hair cut. So a few mornings later I left the apartment for my hair appointment. I hadn't seen Bruno and Rosemary in years, it seemed. I would splurge and go see them at Elizabeth Arden. I started walking down Fifth Avenue, and it reminded me of John walking to his office every morning, smiling at the doormen, saying good morning to them, talking and singing to himself. I did the same thing. A Barry Manilow song called "Day Break" had been on the radio. I even bought the album that has it on it. It is cheerful, upbeat, and I sang it to myself over and over again walking all the way down Fifth Avenue to Elizabeth Arden at 54th Street. But there was a numbness about John; telling Bruno and Rosemary about him seemed too easy. I could practically feel their legs buckling under them with their reaction, but I felt little. Why did I have such a strong inner insistence that I be cheerful? It worried me that I had not faced John's death. I would be the last person in line to tell me this. I had heard it from everyone. I wished I could cry, but I couldn't, I couldn't get out of that cloud of no feeling.

Finally, by the end of February, I was able to take the baby outside. I pushed the carriage to the oval behind the museum where John had watched the little boys play soccer and where last winter we had thrown snowballs at each other. I smiled at everyone I saw walking toward me. At John's most recent checkup Dr. Lazarus had exclaimed what a "well-tended" baby John was. "He's a happy baby and a relaxed one—it's easy to tell just by looking at him." And was I proud.

A week later my mother drove us out to Bridgehampton

for the weekend. It was the first time I had been there since October 9, five months before, almost half a year. That night was only the second time I had slept in that bed without John, but at least I had John III asleep at the foot of my bed in his carriage.

In October I'd looked at John's clothes hoping, praying he'd wear them again, but doubting it. Now it was for real. I went through his drawers and closet. His blue jeans, the Liberty tie I gave him when I first knew him, his yellow linen Bermuda shorts, the red running shorts, the white running shorts with the tear up the side that I sewed up again and again, the Paul Stuart, Abercrombie's and Feron's tennis shorts and shirts, and all those tennis and running socks and headbands and wristbands. I cried. The clothes were packed up and taken by Mom to a clothes-donation box. There were pictures of John and me that I'd never seen before, taken in July, one of us clowning on the beach and another of him and me walking down the beach, his arm around my shoulder.

My mother drove us down to the beach, the baby in the car seat. I had to get used to it, never to see John walk up the steps with chairs, umbrella and cooler, his hat on his head. It was too cold and windy to take a walk with the baby in his Snuggli, so Mom stayed in the car with him while I ran down to the water. The ocean was very rough, with big gray waves. I shouted, "I hate you! Why did you take him away from me?" to the sky, ocean, sand. I tried throwing a stone, and it landed only a few feet away; John could toss one a great distance. Made me mad I couldn't throw. Tried again and again and was terrible, and it made me wonder who was going to teach John how to throw a ball. How could I be Mommy *and* Daddy? But then I stood rigid and still and asked myself, How have you done it, how have you done it these months? What incredible strength I had had: life, sickness, death, birth all in six

months. There was nothing more and never would be for
me to go through that would again take all my courage.

That Sunday there was a profile of Joseph Heller in the
Times Magazine. He said about his father's dying when he
was five years old something like, "I didn't think about
him and not to think about him meant he hadn't existed."
That's what I did; if I didn't think about John and how
much I missed him, then it didn't hurt, and I suppose that
meant I was trying to deny he was dead or had ever lived
for that matter.

The Rossis were not in good shape either. My father-in-
law, in one call talking to me about Workmen's Compensation and a possible lawsuit against Johns-Manville, the
manufacturers of the asbestos sheeting John had worked
with, asked me to be patient with them. That it was so
hard for them. I was too shy to tell him it was hard for me,
too, to throw away his summer clothes. Aunt Linuccia
came for a visit, and she, too, told me, "You lost a husband, but *they* lost a son." Didn't they realize that little
John had lost a *father*? Why and how did that sick compe-
tition of "our grief is worse than yours" start? It was
"worse" for each one of us, and it sure wasn't going to be
easy for John when he was old enough to understand.

I was now being asked by Nightingale friends questions
like "How are you *really*?" Oh, boy. I was not sure I was
looking forward to going back to work there in April.

Three months after John died the worst thing happened. I dreamed that John had come back, alive and
healthy. He was really there in my dream; I was even welcoming him home in the apartment and he met his son. I
really believed what I'd dreamed. And then I heard the
baby waking up and making his soft, please-feed-me
noises, and I woke up. And slowly, dimly and so sadly I
realized it was just a dream, that John hadn't returned,

that he was still indeed dead, and that I was indeed alone without him in the morning.

A week later, however, I felt quite brave and decided to give a dinner party and invite five Bayberries friends. I now saw why John never minded cleaning up at the end of a party—it gives one the chance to reflect quietly on one's blessings.

Even dead, John provided the biggest laugh that night when I told the story of the Colgate alumnus calling him on a fund-raising telethon, and John asking *him* for "twenty-five dollars until Friday." We all talked about him. I knew there might never be another night like that. People would get bored talking about him soon, I could tell, or feel it was strange.

Everyone except the Bayberries group was full of advice for me: that I must go back to work at Nightingale or else I might "get too wrapped up in your son." "You cannot make him your whole life, Nancy." Who had said I would? I was intolerant of this well-meaning advice and felt that the love I had for my son was the most nourishing and positive part of my life. But I knew, too, without being told, that it was necessary to continue my adult friendships and interests.

CHAPTER NINE

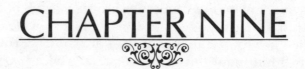

I t seemed that most of the spring was spent remembering
and writing down everything that John liked so that
there'd be a record for his son; I was afraid I was going to
forget what he was like, that I would forget that his
favorite opera was *Boris Godunov* (with Martti Tavela), that
his favorite actor was Joel Grey, that his favorite writers were
all Russian, from Tolstoy and Dostoyevsky to Sholokhov,
Nabokov and Solzhenitsyn, that his favorite thing to eat was
a bowl of homemade soup or Salade Niçoise. And his favorite poets, Tennyson and Pushkin. I went on and on trying to
remember the specifics, afraid that if I didn't remember
every detail, it would somehow mean that I didn't know him
very well or that I already had forgotten him.

I didn't like seeing the trees in Central Park begin to bloom with their pale-green leaves; as I told Esther, I thought spring would help, would make it easier, but instead I was sadder than ever. Yes, she said, spring is rebirth, flowers coming up with new life, and it all just emphasized that John was not there. She told me there was something that she'd like to ask me—did I think John knew he was going to die? I said yes, but that he didn't think it was going to be so soon, that he thought, I think, that he had about a month more. Oh, dear. I hung up with still dumbing, numbing unrealization. Still no raging or tears. I had to make a new life. At least the driving lessons—already I was driving with the trucks on Second Avenue and up and down the FDR Drive—were giving me some confidence, and the recent article about grief in *The New York Times* made me feel less abnormal: that grief is actually the worst for a young widow, that it is even worse than a mother losing a child. It was hard to believe that. But then the article quoted a survey, which said that Americans thought that forty-eight hours to two weeks was enough time "to get over" the loss of an immediate family member. No, it was this four-to-six-month period that was the worst so far. And now reading about the Three Mile Island nuclear accident; a presidential commission had been formed, which included a Middletown, Pennsylvania, housewife and mother of six, to determine how the accident happened and how subsequent confusing and contradictory events and decisions were made. Frightening to think that there might have been a thirteen-year-old boy there who twenty years from now will look as John did in Mt. Sinai. Too, when would a presidential commission be formed to investigate asbestos?

It was right around this time, when my father-in-law had started the necessary legal work to begin a Workmen's Compensation case, that he talked with an old law-school friend who urged him to contact the law firm of Blatt & Fales in Barnwell, South Carolina. He felt that a lawsuit against

Johns-Manville had to be brought. Lawyers at Kelley Drye had mentioned this, too, and had suggested a lawyer who specialized in this kind of legal work. My father-in-law then met with Ron Motley and Terry Richardson from Blatt & Fales, and he was impressed. They met with a few of the partners at Kelley Drye as well, and it was decided that I should retain them.

I didn't expect the complete interest they took in this case and in me. In trying to know me and John better, they asked to see all old photographs of him, our wedding album, and to read all of my diaries. Terry asked if I happened to have taken a photograph of John while he was in the hospital. I looked wide-eyed at him and said, "What? Of course not." Why would anyone want to take a picture of a husband who has mesothelioma? He explained to me how useful such a photograph would have been at the trial, but said that of course he understood why it would never have occurred to me to photograph him when he looked so ill.

Terry asked me about my social life, and I laughed nervously but looked a little shocked as well. It was just too early for me to think of a "social life"; in fact it was an effort to see just about anyone. And I told him about the cocktail party I had forced myself to go to the week before where one couple I'd never met before asked me if I was alone, was my husband with me? "No, I'm a widow," I said. But then I had had to explain how it was that I had a three-month-old son and said, "My husband died in December." Actually, though, I told Terry, having gotten past that, I had a good time, a good time for a widow, that is, not a particularly great time if I'd still been a wife, and I felt more pressure now that I was alone to be charming, smiling and fun. That before I could have leaned back, relaxed and enjoyed watching John glow. Now apparently I had to glow so that I would perhaps be invited back, make new friends, all the ways of behaving I'd hated before I got married. And, too, I told

Terry, the dreams continued, those "He's back, he's really back" dreams, the "I just wanted to wait awhile, Nini, before I came back" dreams.

That spring reminded me of buying life insurance, three different policies. One I got from the savings bank around the corner, and as the man there asked for my doctor's name, address and phone, I thought I'd better call Dr. Uscher's office to say that he might be getting calls from these insurance people. Dr. Uscher answered the phone himself and said he'd been thinking about me and was going "to give me a buzz." He asked how John was, and I told him that Dr. Lazarus at each of his monthly checkups said that he was doing perfectly. Then he asked about me. I told him that I was fine but that sometimes it was rough, that I assumed once I'd gone through the first spring, the first summer, without him that things would be better. Dr. Uscher was happy to hear that I was back at work at Nightingale and that I had such a lovely woman taking care of John. He asked if I had been out to the house, and I told him I went out every weekend, that I was in the process of planting my garden and learning to drive, too. He said, "Good for you. You are fantastic."

It meant a lot to me to hear his praise, feel his silent understanding of what I went through every day. It must have been because his own mother had died of cancer.

The return to work at Nightingale hadn't been as bad as I'd anticipated. For only the first few days—it took about that long for me to see everyone in the building for the "first" time and for them to see me—the awkwardness and gentle compassion in their eyes were almost too much to bear. But then quickly things returned to normal, so much so that the safe, sheltering atmosphere there cocooned me from anything in the real world; I could go about my work there without feeling, and it is now that I look back that I realize the routine—not necessarily the daily contact with people, which is what I was told I needed—that the predictability of the routine there is what I needed then, that that gave me the most necessary sense of "life continues, life goes on." That and the daily routine of caring for John had saved me. He was gaining weight and growing so well.

MAY 1, 1979

Dear Lizzie,

. . . My life is starting to get back to a pretty regular pattern: I come to school in the mornings, stay until 1 p.m., and then go home and play with John in the afternoons. So far it's working out very well, although I can't say I'm accomplishing a great deal at school or doing anything to further a "career," but I think I'm useful to them, and I'm happy to come here. (Even though my baby-sitter makes more than I do, naturally!) I think things will pick up more in the fall when I get more involved in the admissions work. Anyway, it's good to be back here, and it's uncanny how just about nothing has changed—it's as if I haven't had all these months away: R. is still complaining, and everyone else is up to their same old stuff. Incredible. It's very hard for me to take all of what goes on here with great seriousness (the "She didn't turn off the Xerox machine" remarks) in view of what I've been through. That sort of thing seems all the more inconsequential now and really stupid. So, I come and go pretty quietly.

. . . John is thriving. And is so much fun. It sounds like a strange thing to say about one's child, but I'm glad I know him. He has a wonderful personality. He is his own self already at 3½ months—he's not just like John or just like me, but he has his own very definite personality. And I like it.

I don't know how I'd be facing the future without him. Of

course at times it's killing to realize John's not here to share his little accomplishments or to ask questions like "On what side of John's head should I part his hair?" but if I didn't have this little boy, the loneliness and grief would be so much worse. It is so easy to see, Lizzie, how much power a parent has over a child, that one really has the opportunity to affect a child's life dramatically. So, I guess, it's for that reason that I do think it's best for me to go to work and be out of the house for the half-day. I could so easily make John my only reason for living, my only companion, and he could so easily become too dependent on me. It's a very fine line, and I just hope I'm doing the right thing and that I am being a good mother. I do wish that he saw more men. He lives in such a female environment with me and the baby-sitter during the week and in the country with my mother and me on the weekends. However, one of his baby-sitters is a teenage boy, who is fantastic. John loves him, and laughs and kicks whenever he's there.

. . . Please give my best to Woody. I wish you both weren't quite so far away! Sometime, though, I may throw the budget out the window and give you a telephone call. I do miss you.

Much love,
Nancy

As much as I had hated the spring, it was summer I dreaded the most. I could not imagine myself out at that Bridgehampton house in the summer with the baby and my parents. It had been too easy to let my mother take over, even during the spring weekends, and I was starting to resent it. Without John there to humor her, her bossiness and certainty that she knew what was right for both me and the baby were suffocating if understandable. She must have thought that if what had happened to me had happened to her, she would not have been able to cope, so she and my father had the tendency to assume that I could not manage without them. But, although it took all my courage, I went with them out there for Memorial Day weekend, the first without John.

It was a weekend of frantic buying. I hadn't done anything like that ever before: I bought tomato plants for the garden, a bicycle for myself and a painting at a gallery, "Lobelia," by Nancy Wissemann-Widrig. It looks just like Bayberries' front-porch rail with Georgica Pond beyond, clouded in mist, as it was in the mornings during our honeymoon in 1974. The best part of the weekend was meeting the woman who owned the gallery. Her husband had died of cancer in 1971. And between us there was a silent understanding of the loss, the awfulness, helplessness, aching heart and loneliness, all in a moment of silence. That she had remarried made me smile.

But the next weekend was worse. I was proud of myself that I triumphantly, although expensively, got through Memorial Day weekend, but I could not maintain it, and on the following Saturday I bicycled over to Bayberries, thinking maybe that would make me feel better; I had to see that house again. I pedaled up the driveway. No cars. I knocked on the door. No answer. I cautiously turned the door handle and it opened. The old familiar smell of a musty house that has been open only a couple of weeks since being closed up for the winter the previous autumn rushed to my face. The yellow dining room to the right, the dark-wood living room to the left, the green staircase in front of me, which went to "our" room. I called out hello, hello. No, no one was there, not Alvin from the new generation of Kelley Drye lawyers who now rented the house, not anybody. I walked first to the kitchen. There was the same kitchen table, the dishwasher that hooked up to the faucet in the sink, the same tea kettle. Next to it was the washer and dryer the owners had put in for us that first summer. The pantry was the same, even the same odd assortment of jelly glasses and wineglasses, the same dishes and plates. Same books in the bookcases in the living room, same plant stand and hanging plant holder in the side sunroom. And then up the stairs, the funny Egyptian-looking fabric wallpaper, the window seat at the top of the staircase, and there to the left was our room, the pink room. And its bathroom with the same shower curtain that David and John put up over the bathtub when they installed a shower head. Guessed this was Alvin's room now. I recognized a lot of his stuff. But maybe not, as when I went into David and Carolyn's room, I thought I saw a suit of his hanging in that closet. The other bedrooms, the little maid's room, then upstairs to the attic with the two tiny bedrooms up there, the blue one that we all painted, the tub with feet and the old sink, the cedar smell coming from the locked cedar closets. The old clothes hooks on one wall where I'd hung herbs to dry one summer so long ago.

I walked down the stairs in a daze and out the front door and closed it behind me and walked down over the lawn to the little spot of sand on Georgica Pond. I sat down and stared out over the pond. There were no words. I'd forgotten so many things, so many pieces of furniture, and I had thought, I told myself, that I had it and each moment remembered so well. And he was gone forever. It was somebody else's house now. It would never be mine. But at least there was the comfort of sitting on the same sand we used to sit on together, looking up at the moon on summer nights. This place knew him, and that would never leave.

But it also meant that I had to get away that summer. I couldn't stand the thought of spending July, John's and my vacation month, with my mother that year. Right then

I started thinking about going to Maine or Vermont with the baby.

Even baseball that summer didn't help. I watched Tom Seaver, then with Cincinnati, pitch against the Astros one night. After he gave up a walk, allowing the tying run to advance to third, he looked down at his feet, and a drop of sweat rolled down and off his nose. Just like John. John so sweaty and dripping after tennis or running, saying, "Give me a kiss." Tom Seaver so much like John: looks, manner, everything. I used to tell John that he was an even handsomer Tom Seaver; he liked that. In a way, now seeing Seaver and watching him get older was like seeing Bunky at his age. Then Seaver got taken out of the game, not very happy about it, pretty revved up, and as he walked to the dugout, he wiped his face with the front of his shirt—that really was just like John. I had to get out of there that summer.

It became clearer in the following days that it was not only Long Island I had to get away from, but also my family and friends. I had to take my baby to a part of the world I'd never been to, but even more important, to a part of the world John had never rested a foot on. I couldn't bear to go to a place that had once welcomed a John Rossi, to a place where, even worse, he and I had been in love together. I had to do something on my own, something so dramatic that I would, from the sheer courage it took me to do such a thing, as a result find confidence and comfort within myself.

But where could I go? I had some money from the law firm. I could use it for psychiatry, which I didn't feel I needed because here I was every day proving that I was coping by going to work in the admissions office at Nightingale and by taking care of my son. Or I could use some of that money for an extravagant gift to myself, for an adventure, for a journey that might give me the guts to go on living. So many fears to conquer on a journey like that: planes to begin with, which I hated; being completely responsible for my little boy in a strange place; even meeting new people without the security of John there beside me. I chose the latter, but I had no idea of where to go. I knew I had to be in a country that had first-rate medical services in case the baby got sick and in a country whose language I knew. But before even considering England, France or Italy, I received in the mail an unsolicited advertisement, addressed to Mr. and Mrs. Rossi, inviting us to visit a resort in Wyoming, under the same management as one John and I had traveled to in the Virgin Islands.

Wyoming. Even then it sounded magical, just the name of the state. Even though I'd gone to school in Boulder, Colorado, I'd never gotten up to Wyoming, and my closest connection to it was knowing the roommate of a friend of mine in Boulder who had grown up in Cheyenne. I recalled that my mother's mother's sister had been the first of the Nichols women to build a life out in Colorado, and, with her dimly in my mind, I'd followed by going to college there, but my conscious thought now was that Nichols women go west. And that I was going to Wyoming, to a state no one in my family had ever been to.

A call out there confirmed that because of the summer of '79 gas crisis, they'd had some cancellations and that, yes, they would have a cabin for me and for my five-month-old son and that, yes, they not only allowed but enjoyed children as guests. Then I called the airlines. Yes, I could get a reservation at such short notice. And then I called two friends from my University of Colorado days. Why, yes, they'd love to see me and the baby when we passed through Denver on our way back to New York. It was so easy to arrange that I said yes at every turn and wound up realizing a few days later that within a week

John and I were going to Wyoming! To the mountains! Whence cometh my help. Maybe God was out there.

We got up at five-thirty and I fed the baby and got him dressed and ready for the car that would pick us up at seven. We were almost the only ones on the road as we sped to Kennedy Airport. The city looked still and quiet that hot, smoggy summer morning as I looked back at it from the Triboro Bridge. There was no turning back. We were going to Wyoming. The flying was fine, the landing in Denver fine; the changing to the Frontier Airlines flight was not fine. They didn't have our reservation. Frontier was happy to refund my tickets and get us on the next plane, though. It would leave five hours from then for Jackson, Wyoming.

At last we boarded the old Constellation prop plane. Seats about thirty, I would guess. John on my lap. It was at least a two-hour flight. We landed in Jackson, the Tetons rising out of nothing into the sky like church spires. Our luggage had gone ahead on the other plane, and here it was in this tiny little airport piled onto an outdoor wooden table. A bus took us to Jenny Lake. It was nine at night, but it was only just getting dark, and as we pulled out of the one airport driveway, the Tetons were back in view. I'd made the right decision.

Jenny Lake Lodge contained a small hotel desk, the hotel's one telephone, a small lounge and the dining room, still busy with those eating their dinners. I signed in and very quickly realized the place was staffed by young college students. As we checked in, the manager told me they'd been looking forward to our arrival and that he had a nice surprise. He was putting me and John into a two-room bedroom/living-room suite cabin for the same rate as what our single cabin would have been. He knew I was a widow, his own wife's first husband had died, too, and he wanted me to have the best time I could here. The wheelbarrow carrying our luggage went ahead of us, the flashlight the boy carried lighting our way on the paths. Towering pine trees surrounded us. The smell was perfume.

Then there we were; he unlocked the door and turned on the outdoor porch lights and the lights inside and stepped aside to let me enter. John was peering over my shoulder as I held him to me. Had I eaten dinner? the boy asked. No? He'd send dinner over to me. There was an ice bucket and a small refrigerator. I put some ice cubes in a glass and filled it up with water. The young man returned with dinner and also a crib, which he set up in the bedroom. I changed John into his sleep suit and he went right to sleep. I ate and then stepped outside onto the porch. It had gotten quite cold; the stars were brilliant and the moon bright. I looked up at the sky and said to myself, "I did it, Bunky, I really did it!"

The next morning after breakfast I put John in the stroller and we took a long walk to String Lake. He had his morning nap in an alpine meadow. I'd never seen such flowers: red Indian paintbrush, scarlet gentian, bluebell, columbine, larkspur, wild roses, glacier lily, lupine, cornflower. A rainbow of reds, yellows, purples and blues and carpets of fragrant sagebrush.

The afternoon we spent just resting and napping, and in the evening we went in for dinner, John sitting in his stroller by my chair. We were invited to join the table of a couple from Chicago who had spoken to me at lunch. But soon it was clear I was with a couple who couldn't stand to be by themselves and had to have others to talk to. Even though John slept through most of dinner, it was exhausting making conversation with these people and at the same time making sure John was okay. When he woke up, he fussed, and the wife asked to hold him while I ate, but I wish I could have enjoyed the delicious trout more. Then

John was passed to another woman at a table next to ours. It was too much. I tried to be gay and carefree about it, but the fact was I didn't like him or me being with this very rowdy, unhappy couple, and I was glad when dinner was over and we went back to our cabin.

The next day John and I returned to String Lake, and a young man walked by with his camera, and I asked him if he'd do me a big favor and take a picture of John and me with my camera. I had so few photographs of the two of us together. He said sure and had us stand in the sun with the lake and mountains behind us. He took the picture and then joked that he would send me his bill. I liked that. This very friendly Western attitude was something to try to take back to New York with me. I went swimming. It was glorious. Such a clear lake, it was easy to see the bottom. As I swam farther out into the lake, John resting with a little girl watching over him on his blanket on the shore, I saw a father plunge into the water while his children giggled and squealed, "Daddy, Daddy!" But instead of it making me sad, my immediate thought was that one day I'd be back here with a man John would call Daddy.

After dinner that night, John asleep in his crib, I went on a bike ride to the "Cathedral" lookout spot on the main road. As I got there, I looked to my left and was about to get off the bike to enjoy the view at dusk when fifty feet away from me was a moose! He was munching the grasses and sage, and I pretended to turn the bike around calmly and head back. He looked up at me, and I probably did exactly the wrong thing: I pedaled as fast as I could back to the cabin.

One afternoon the college girl who cleaned the cabin baby-sat for John while I went bike riding for two hours. I was a little nervous about going so far, but curiosity propelled me all the way to Jenny Lake itself. By the time I got there, it was gray, cloudy and wild windy. I walked on some of the trails around and down by the shore of the lake and took some pictures. The next morning I walked John back over to Jenny Lake in his stroller. Three miles. We sat on a rock, he in my lap, looking at the lake in the brilliant sun. Today I could see, with the bright-blue sky overhead, why it was called the "blue jewel" of the Tetons. The day before it had looked like dull pewter.

As John and I were sitting there, people in a camper from Montana began talking to me—they had, they said, a grandson exactly the same age as John, born January 24. They said then that "Grandpa died January nineteenth—so we lost a life, but we gained a life in the family." I said the same thing happened to me except that it was my husband. They looked stricken. What I had been through, and I could still talk about it. Someday, however, I may never, ever be able to say one word about this tragedy or ever refer to it. I may become like Theodore Roosevelt, who forbade any mention in his presence of his Alice, his first wife who died when they were so young.

I was still shy with the other guests. It was more fun to talk to the college kids and ask them where they were in school and what they were studying and how they managed to land such great summer jobs. The dreams here, though, were too vivid, more vivid than those in New York; the mountain air stimulated my imagination to dreams of hospitals and IVs and cancer.

Our week was over. The last night I sat outside in one of the rockers on the porch. My life really was going to be all right. I'd done that trip on my own; I had found there was joy in new experiences, not fear. Those mountains were my church. I wasn't sure that I had found any answers there, any hows and whys of John's death, but I was going to continue to live, that much I knew.

CHAPTER TEN

It was September again, and I was losing my Wyoming hopefulness. I felt more alone in New York City than in Wyoming. John's last birthday had been a year ago. Our last anniversary a year ago. His operation a year ago. I couldn't help myself; I relived each day of the last year over and over again. The highlight of October was that at my six-month checkup with Dr. Uscher he asked me whom I was dating, was there just one? Very funny. I felt as if my legs had been frozen. And then the news that the pregnancy had cleared up the infertility problem. I looked at him blankly, stunned. I couldn't even say anything. I didn't believe it.

I called him the next day to make sure that I'd heard him correctly and that I correctly understood the implications of what he'd said. Yes, he said, I certainly now did have to worry about birth control. He said, "I tried to slip that in." I said, "I am really dense." He said, "I know." After all these years. Shit. I couldn't believe it. "Come in," he said, "and we'll fit you with a diaphragm." I told him I'd let him know when, that it might be a long time, as "I don't even *know* anyone."

And John not here to take advantage of this good news so that we could have more children. I was furious. This was the final unfairness. These autumn days were making me bitter. What bitterness and resentment I felt toward healthy young men in their lovely suits, shirts and ties and with headfuls of beautiful hair and smiles on their faces and an expectant briskness to their walk. I had to close my eyes when I walked on packed sidewalks full of them.

MONDAY, OCTOBER 8, 1979

Dear Lizzie,

. . . The trip to the Grand Tetons in Wyoming was an outstanding success, and if I weren't so conventional, I might even seriously act on a tremendous urge to move out there. Instead I feel as if I've found a private place to which John and I will return in the summers and the memories of which will get me through the long winter days. The physical beauty of those mountains was magical, spiritual, and so full of hope. Sounds strange I guess how a place, rather than a person, can overwhelm one so much and give one the same reassurance and faith that a person could give. I don't know, but I left there feeling so optimistic about my future and capabilities. And that optimism carried me through getting my driver's license (at last!) and now seems to give me courage as I drive in and out of NYC to Bridgehampton alone, with John in his car seat. It is so satisfying to be able to go out to the house with John (just the two of us) and plant bulbs and walk on the beach.

School is very much the same except more crowded! Because I still am on the same schedule I had last spring, I get home by 1:30 and have the afternoons with John. On Wednesdays though I keep Aloma all day, and I go to the movies! It's a great time of day, and I have the theater usually to myself, and afterward I take a long walk. People have suggested that I go to museums instead, but not only does my brain seem not up to it, I've always found it hard to go to a museum alone—much more fun with someone else.

One thing I look forward to with a mixture of pleasure and reluctance is the beginning of my subscription to the opera which I've treated myself to. The first time will be the worst, as I've not been in the opera house since John died, and that building seemed almost as much a part of our marriage as our apartment, but at least the first opera is a funny one (The Barber of Seville), so that should help. You know how much I loved going, so I'm forcing myself not to give up going.

Things are otherwise going pretty well. John's pediatrician and my ob-gyn man, that Dr. Uscher, both think I should be out dating up a storm! Who with? I've gotten to the point where I wouldn't mind going out to dinner and talking with someone, but whether it's today or next year doesn't seem to matter to me. I guess I'm finally getting used to and settled in my new life with this baby, and that's enough work right there. It's the talking with and being in the same room with a man I miss, but I don't miss that mad scramble of dating, phone calls.

I try my best not to wrap myself up in John's life, but it's not easy. He is the reason I can even exist, and his humor and now his curiosity fill my days with smiles. I push him on the swings in the park, he's just starting to stand, everything is new to him, and it seems such a privilege to be guiding and teaching him. He is starting to talk and says Dada (!) all the time, which used to unnerve me, but it seems to be the first sound all babies make, and then a few weeks ago he finally started calling me Mama. Of course that made me fly. As I keep reminding myself, even though it's a life I never expected for myself and is so different from most people's, it's a life I've

gotten used to and really like, so that it seems unusual or
pitiful only to others, not to myself anymore. . . .

Love,
Nancy

When vivid memories of John and of events that once
happened, of things we used to do together and of places
we were together, came upon me unexpectedly, my throat
constricted, I couldn't swallow. It wasn't really "a lump in
the throat," but more like my throat was drying up and
actually starting to ache, and then that aching worked its
way up to my eyes, and my eyes half closed in pain, and
as a result of that my nose pinched and flared and my
mouth became pursed, as if eating something sour, more
sour than lemons, more like a bitter sensation, a sensation
of bitter, dried, useless herbs, and my forehead wrinkled,
the shoulders stiffened, and the neck tightened, but the
rest of me was like jelly; only from the shoulders up was I
in paralyzed constriction. And then it was over. The memory that had hurt so because of its vividness of past happy
times had faded and gone away. Life was back to the now,
to the normal.

In late October I decided to telephone the office where
Drew, a man I had seen before I knew John, worked. I had
met him one day when he came downtown to have lunch
with his college roommate, who worked at Merrill Lynch,
where I was then a secretary. He was an officer at the
Rockefeller Center branch of a New York bank. In the two
years Drew and I saw each other, he became a trusted,
dear friend, and although it became clear we would not
marry, we continued once a year to call and write each
other to share good news or sad. He answered the phone
himself that October day; he knew, he said, from the
sound of my voice that I was about to tell him something
important, but he surely wasn't prepared to hear of John's

death. I told him I would like to see him, to talk to him, and could we meet for lunch? "Oh, my God," he said, "of course, Nance, of course." And we made a date for lunch in November.

I began looking forward so much to seeing him, because I felt he was the only person in front of whom I could break down. I realized that it had been like planning a war, being a general, organizing thousands of troops: first facing John's cancer, making sure everyone behaved in front of him as he wanted, screening calls, visits, hearing of his death, organizing his cremation, service, being the stoic strong widow, being the superhuman mother as I gave birth to our son alone, months of devoted care of my little boy, the ease I showed the world, going back to work, too. How had I done it? And never once breaking down in front of others. Instead, always cheery, always showing hope and ability in front of others. Oh, I'd certainly cried to myself, alone. But, God, I'd longed for a person who could understand, who would hold me and let me cry. It was not fair, I guess, to ask Drew to do this, to give this of himself, but he was the only one I felt comfortable enough with: with him the general could put down her sword, could cry, could be comforted. He was, in many ways, one of the dearest friends of my life.

One evening, as I was walking up to Rodd and Janet's, I saw a couple I knew through the window of a bar. I waved to them, and they waved for me to come in. I had a glass of wine with them while they waited for their friends to show up, and while we were talking, a man standing next to me said, "Oh, my God, I've fallen in love." And then to the man he was with, "She's beautiful." My friends and I looked at each other with questioning raised eyebrows. It took me a while before I realized he was talking about me. His conversation to his companion was loud, about the opera, and he was standing so near me that with me on the bar stool my head must have been under his arm, with him able to look at me without my being able to see him. I wish now I'd had the courage to turn and smile perhaps, but I was paralyzed, remembering unconsciously, I think, John's opening hello to me: "Hi, I'm John. You're the most beautiful girl I've ever seen in my life." I felt bad because I didn't do anything to acknowledge I'd even *heard* that man's nice words. Instead, I ignored them. Shyness and tentativeness like that would not bring friends—men— into my life, but I just couldn't help myself.

I began entertaining. One night I made a wonderful chili dinner for fourteen. But I still dreamed sad dreams of John. I remembered exactly how he'd looked a year before: those swollen legs and feet and thin arms. Somehow what was starting to fade in my memory was the hugeness of his stomach. I hadn't noticed it then, and I didn't vividly remember it now. That ravaged body. We truly, in our silent, all-loving way, took care of each other and each other's spirits during those last weeks we had. It may not have been other people's way of dealing with cancer and death, but it was ours. And our quiet understanding and presence needed no words. We were one person in marriage and particularly then, and I guess that's why I could still feel Bunky and his strength alive in me. We adored each other and how we complemented each other—he breezy and outgoing and me sensitive to others' feelings and so admiring of the wonderful joy he got from each day, from being alive. We were the perfect couple, not only to the world but to ourselves. How happy we were, and I have the most precious memories. I am lucky. And to be blessed with our little boy. John had seen to it all.

I listened to as many Wagner recordings as I could get. I used to hate his music, but I now appreciated that he understood, his music clearly understands, life's emotions. I listened to Birgit Nilson sing the "Liebestode" on the car's cassette deck over and over when I drove down to the beach.

One day in the kitchen an anger and fury so consumed me that afterward I felt maybe now I could begin to come out of the darkness. It was as if my fingers and toes had become talons, hideous claws, and I jumped up and down, a hideous moan racking my throat, fierce and rigid, bent over, wailing. And I kept jumping up and down. I was no longer controlled by valued, tempered emotions, but was an animal, a primitive lonely soul, crying out in anger and loss for her beloved. The loss I had endured, the pain my son would one day have to bear upon hearing of his father's death, the bravery of my husband for me, it all came crashing down. And I, alone in my beloved kitchen, could keep this firecracker display of grief and rage subdued no longer. Perhaps now some light would begin to shine for me. A return to the real world.

I had to allow the passage of time to decide whether or not my lunch with Drew was positive or negative. I obviously had been hoping for so much and found his brisk probing of my emotional state unsettling. I was not ready to have the privacy of my emotions scrutinized. I left having the horrible suspicion I'd disappointed him—perhaps my looks, what I talked about—I don't know. He looked so much the same to me and as physically desirable as in the old days. I was fully aware the past couldn't be repeated, but I was hoping for a new foothold. Perhaps it was for the best; perhaps I was deserving of more than that friendship could offer. It was just that I felt so comfortable with him, regardless of the fact that he made me as nervous as hell for the first part of the lunch.

I finally got the courage to call Dr. Uscher's office about the feeling that there was no one I could talk to, that what I'd been through was so unique that there were no others from whom I could ask advice. I asked his secretary, Ann, for him to call me when he had a few quiet moments during the week. He called back that night, and I asked him if he knew anyone who had dealt with people who had lost a . . . (my voice drifted off), not a psychiatrist who wanted to talk about my childhood. He said he knew what I meant, and that he would ask around. He said he realized these next couple of months were going to be just as rough as the first ones. A few days later he gave me the name of Dr. Ivan Goldberg; his specialty was death, the grief and mourning process. Sounded perfect. I made an appointment to see him.

His office was right around the corner from Nightingale. He was a bear of a man, well over six feet, with a beard and a fine smile. I spent an incredible hour with him. I wasn't nuts after all. It is "worse" as the one-year mark approaches. Very normal in the grief process. Keep up that diary, he said. In fact, in later sessions he thought that perhaps Columbia-Presbyterian or, really, I guess, Columbia University Press might be interested in publishing it, that it would be very helpful to other families, other patients, other hospitals. But maybe, he mused, just from what I'd told him about it, maybe it might have a broader appeal. Did I know anyone in publishing who could take a look at it? Yes, Julie Houston, a girl I grew up with. Fine, he said. Show it to her.

I went home and read and reread my diaries from the year before, and each day was described in detail. I could not talk. I was alone and felt abandoned. No one could imagine what I'd been through, what I'd demanded of myself. I felt weak and numb.

My Diary:

FRIDAY, NOVEMBER 30, 1979

On the eve of John's baptism I ask Bunky that he help me in the years ahead to bring up our son to be a proud man and a kind man, a man in fact like Bunky. I want my son to be respected and loved by all the men and women in his life. I want him to prize honesty and gentle humor and generosity as the strengths given to only the strongest of men. I know the spirit of his father will help him accomplish the important tasks and requirements his life will demand of him, whether they be academic, physical, spiritual or humanistic. Even at ten months of age, I am certain my son will become a great man. And the thing that pleases me most is that he will do it on his own.

THURSDAY, DECEMBER 6, 1979

It hurts so much that I find I cannot write in here, in this diary. So soon it will be one year. Everything is crowded out of my mind except my memories of Bunky. Cruelly, every night he is in my dreams. So softly and feebly I cry, "I want him back," knowing the impossibility. Our son fills up so much and gives me so much joy, and yet the empty space of where my Bunky was is immense. My darling, how will I cope with the awful reality of Dec. 17th? Our first year apart.

SATURDAY, DECEMBER 15, 1979

Same as last year, incredible: Aida *is the Saturday opera from the Metropolitan;* Miracle on 34th Street *is on TV in the evening. But this year at least I'm writing Christmas cards and enclosing pictures of my boy. And I bought a wreath and Christmas-tree lights today. And I know that somehow I'll get through these next days. I'll relive every moment, from the phone call of John's death through the service through the birth of our son. It is so cruel. How can he be dead one year? Will I ever stop crying for him? And yet somehow I feel Bunky's arms around my shoulders tonight, and I remember him saying a year ago, "Take care of yourself, Nini."*

SUNDAY, DECEMBER 16, 1979

I feel crushed. How can I live through tomorrow? The worst day of my life. Bless you, Bunky. Take care. And give me strength not to collapse and break down tomorrow. I can't believe you've been gone a year already.

MONDAY, DECEMBER 17, 1979

This morning I bathed our little boy and fed him his oatmeal cereal with applesauce and gave him some orange juice.

AFTER MIDNIGHT

"The nerves sit ceremonious like tombs."
I have not even cried today, not even walking down Park Avenue at 11 p.m. on my way home from the book-club meeting, where we discussed Philip Roth's Ghost Writer. *When will it come pouring out?*
At least today was bright and sunny although bitterly cold—not the gray, sad day of John's death. My darling.

WEDNESDAY, DECEMBER 19, 1979

John, one year ago, cremated today. Burned. Ashes to ashes. Awful. My poor darling sick man.

LATER

A hideous cab driver in the snow, wanting to date me, me saying no, a widow, and him telling me my husband's death was "God's will." Shit. If I ever hear that garbage again from anyone, I will puke!

FRIDAY, DECEMBER 21, 1979

Last night a cocktail party, and after I leave I walk down to Park, over to Madison, down Madison, up Madison, and

decide to see if Jack Garraty [a Kelley Drye friend] is home.
He is, and we sit and drink his scotch and talk and talk.
And do even more important talking at Bailiwick over a
glass of wine. Wonderful laughter out of him when I tell
him that I've always thought a certain fellow at Kelley Drye
smelled like old cheese. He tells me about his current women
problems.

LATER

I feel like sitting quietly and trying to remember and re-
enjoy every moment of last night. To be able to talk to some-
one, to have Jack listen, I am flying. Him showing me his
apartment and the things that are special to him: his paint-
ings, his grandmother's furniture, photograph of his best
friend, lending me the Ansel Adams book and others, find-
ing out he graduated from Collegiate in '67! Talking about
painting, writing, things that I love, things I haven't talked
about with anyone, even my John, for years. Him telling me
that fleeting relationships don't cause any personal happi-
ness, even selfish pleasure, that men are forced through peer
pressure to pursue one-night stands and that they don't
really like it! Never knew that. I mean, I knew that sort of
life isn't a man's ideal, but I somehow thought that they
didn't dislike it so much. Me telling him I am too contained
and he thinking I am open and easy with words. I then told
him how I used to love to go to parties with John because I
could relax and observe everyone enjoying John's jokes and
happy, funny manner. Jack telling me that now being forced
to talk and make my own way is not all bad at all.

I tried to explain my love of Wyoming. That after months
of hearing things like John's death was God's will and that
he now has found peace, that those mountains were the only
things that made any sense, that from them, from nature, I
began to come to terms with John's death and perhaps began
to understand what my new life was going to be like. I doubt

that even those mountains will help me forgive his death
or believe that there was any meaning to it, except that it
was fucking chance, a zillion-to-one shot, and it had to be
Bunky.

LATER

It's like breathing and laughing and being alive—I can't
stop. What hope last night gave me—for myself, for all the
fine young men left in the world who are alive, even though
John's dead. I no longer want them dead, too; I want them
all alive, and I want to meet as many as possible. There's
not a man in the world who today can intimidate me or
make me feel shy or awkward, and that's because I have my
son, and men are just my dear boy grown up. All those
years before John of fright and nervousness and self-
consciousness about them were a waste. I think I can now
risk meeting another. I'd become so comfortable in the safety
and security of John's love, but now that I have to be on my
own again, I think I can be more confident about myself
than in those single years before our marriage.

SUNDAY, DECEMBER 23, 1979

It's hard to believe that the anniversary of John's death
will always be exactly a week before Christmas Eve. That
week is so long somehow; it seems like two weeks instead of
one have passed since last Monday and the 17th.

I look forward to my boy's first Christmas. What work I
have put into it. I can't wait to read him The Night Before
Christmas tomorrow night, hang up his stocking, leave
cookies and milk for Santa, fill his stocking, and arrange the
presents under the tree. I can be Mommy and Daddy for as
long as necessary.

CHRISTMAS EVE
DECEMBER 24, 1979

I never thought a year ago that a year later I'd be sitting

next to a toy truck for my son, having already read him The Night Before Christmas, *hung up his stocking, and poured milk and set out two Christmas cookies for Santa. I can't say I'm totally happy—I miss Bunky with great hurt—but at least I'll be smiling this year when I see my dearest boy play with his new toys. I am blessed to have him.*

CHRISTMAS MORNING
DECEMBER 25, 1979

At 7:20 I go into John's room, where I hear him making his morning soft-talking sounds. I turn on the light and show him his filled stocking. He sees the furry Santa Claus sticking out of the top and smiles and laughs and reaches for it. I then take him in my arms, with him holding the stocking, and we go sit in my bed, as Sandy and I used to do with Mom and Dad, to open the presents. He loves the music box that goes by pulling the cord that Granny found for him and Dad's baseball bat, and the squeaky bath toys. John gets so excited about the toys, the tissue paper and red ribbon, that while he sits on my bed, he hugs everything he can reach to him and kicks his feet back and forth. Pure joy. Smiling and laughing. A long day ahead of us, but we'll be all right. My dearest boy.

NEW YEAR'S EVE/NEW YEAR'S DAY
1:30 A.M. JANUARY 1, 1980

Tonight the first night I go out without my wedding rings. I feel not even half whole without them. Don't know how long I can keep them off.

I force myself to go to Victor and Claire's party at 49 East 86th Street. As I stand by the long windows on the 17th floor, looking out at the fireworks over Central Park, with their other guests, midnight chimes. All around me couples are kissing, toasts to their life in the '80s are given to each other. I am solitary, somehow encased in glass, and simply and not even sadly observing what is going on around me. It is a crystal-clear night with a full moon, the window panes are gleaming and lights on Christmas trees from other terraces are reflected. I see a brilliant star above, as good as seeing a seagull, and I feel it is John. I sent my love up to that star, and I, quietly in my mind, while the others are reacting to the new decade, tell him I love him.

Through Jack Garraty's brotherly, concerned friendship I began to get the courage to go to parties, to be able to go into a restaurant with friends. And a year later, when Drew and I met again, he gave me the confidence necessary to accept blind dates, but as I told him, the young men I do meet are awkward around me, saying things like "My divorce was awful, but it can't have been as bad as what happened to you. How did you live through it? You must be a very strong person." It is hard work, I told Drew, making others at ease when they hear what has happened to me for the first time, and I wish all of the questions about one's past that people on a first date do ask each other were not allowed until maybe the third date.

One thing I noticed immediately that was different from my dating him and others before I married John is that eight years later we all have so much more baggage of life experience weighing us down. As a twenty-two-year-old, the main questions one is asked are where are you working, what do you do? And where did you go to school? At thirty-one the questions I was asked were are you divorced, do you have any children? And it was always that question "Are you divorced?" that stopped my tongue. The man could tell that I had paused and he had to wonder why I couldn't answer, but I was trying to find the perfect phrase to say, "No, I'm a widow," or "No, my husband died two years ago," something that didn't land with such a thud on a restaurant table or on the floor of a crowded cocktail party. A friend suggested I say, "No, I'm not married," but that didn't work either, because then they would say, "Have you ever been married?" and there I would be again. That's why it was easier to be around people who knew me before John died—I didn't have to explain anything to them.

But in a perverse way I didn't particularly want to date anyone who knew me and John well; talk to them, yes, but not date them. Too, most of the blind dates my friends arranged for me were with lawyers, so that meant their asking if there was a lawsuit under way, and when I told them yes, that a lawsuit had been filed against Johns-Manville, that at this point it was just a matter of occasionally signing medical release forms, that managed to take up the rest of the evening's talk. And then they got away fast. Being a widow is not exactly a turn-on for men, I told Drew.

"Jesus, kid," Drew said, "I hadn't thought about that. Look, let's have lunch next week. Is Wednesday good for you? You've got someone to take care of John, right? Okay, well, I'll make a reservation at our old restaurant for twelve-thirty then. Take it easy, kid, we'll have a good talk."

I'd forgotten all about that restaurant. The last time I had been there with him had been sort of a farewell lunch, to tell him that I was going to marry John Rossi. Even though we'd stopped seeing each other after John and I started dating, I, a year and a half later, wanted to see him again and say goodbye, and he wanted to as well.

That Wednesday I remember I stepped nervously out of the cab and walked through the same doors and, as it turned out, to practically the same table to say hello to Drew again. He was the one who remembered that we were seated so near "our" table; I'd forgotten. But what I remembered very quickly, within minutes of looking and scanning his face, was how happy being around him made me feel. It wasn't at all like the lunch a year before at that sterile restaurant near Rockefeller Center. I was smiling so much that when I raised the glass of wine he'd ordered for me to my lips, I missed, spilling a bit of it over myself. "Oh, how I've missed that," he said. "Same old Nancy. We can dress you up but we can't take you out." He laughed. Then he went ahead—actually remembered—and ordered exactly what we had eaten for lunch there the last time. I'd really just wanted to see him again, to talk to him, to reaffirm a friendship in the midst of reestablishing myself as an independent woman, although now with a child to raise by myself, and here he was practically courting me. I wasn't prepared for the gentleness, the understanding that overcame me by waves from his side of the table.

A glass of wine with our lunch, some coffee with our dessert, and almost three hours later it was time to leave. He had to get back to the office; I back to the baby-sitter and John. We walked the fifteen blocks back to his office, and in front of the building he waved for a taxi for me; one stopped, and, running into his arms, skipping high on my feet, I met his face and kissed him goodbye. We glanced around and saw that the people who had witnessed this were smiling. My face red and overcome by my own audaciousness, I quickly climbed into the cab. He closed the door and waved.

I remember I leaned back in the taxi and closed my eyes and felt how lucky I'd been that I'd had the chance to tell him everything: about John, about mesothelioma, about asbestos, about Johns-Manville and the lawsuit, about being tired of doing everything with my son alone, about blind dates, about being the odd number at dinner parties, and that he understood and still considered me one of his best friends. This quiet, euphoric silence lasted about five blocks in the slow-moving traffic up Park Ave-

nue when the cab driver began talking. Talking about
Yosemite camping trips, about moving from San Francisco
to New York, about becoming a cab driver here and how
girls at bars here drop him and freeze up once they ask
and he tells them that he's a cab driver. He told about one
experience in particular when at the Lone Star Café he was
speaking to a girl at the bar and unbeknown to him she
had a boyfriend, who upon approaching the two of them
and seeing them chatting, pushed him up against the wall
and "busted three of my ribs." I said, "You mean he broke
them?" I'd woken from my romantic revery and was
amazed and disgusted. He talked more about New York,
how very different it is from the West, and I began nodding in agreement, and began to join his nonstop conversation, especially when he explained that he meant the
Rocky Mountains and Grand Tetons West in comparison
to New York, not the "Coast" West of California. I was by
now so absorbed in the conversation that I'd forgotten
Drew. I told the cab driver that my son and I had been to
the Grand Tetons, twice in fact, and that I had gone to
college in Colorado.

That was all he needed to hear, and he was off telling
stories of hang-gliding with his brother out there, of pan-
ning for gold with his brother, and how they subsequently
sold their "staking land," at his brother's insistence, for
$1,200 only to know now that it was one of the largest
areas of gold production. "I shouldn't always listen to my
brother!" Then I told him, regarding hang-gliding, adven-
tures, taking chances, that one must do them, *if* one en-
joys them, and take the risk because one never knows
what's around the corner, and I blurted out, stupidly,
really now robbing the afternoon of its fairyland quality,
that I had found survival in taking chances, in having ad-
ventures, since my husband so unexpectedly died. The
cab driver turned around and looked at me—I was thinking he had to be my age or a year older—and his eyes were

filling with tears as he brought out his wallet and opened it to a photograph of a young woman. "That was my wife. She died eight years ago. She was learning to fly a plane and had an accident. She left me with our four-month-old daughter. I've always wanted to believe that she died happy, happy because she was doing something that gave her pleasure."

Oh, God, I thought. He knows. We both knew. He behind that bulletproof plastic shield, and me, the passenger, on the other side.

"I've never remarried," he said, "have you?"

"Oh, no," I said as I shook my head from side to side.

He then ripped a piece of paper, wrote his name and telephone number on it. "I know where you're coming from," he said. "If you ever want to call and just talk, I'll understand."

And not knowing what I could do for him, when a hug is prevented by the plastic bulletproof shield, I gave him eight dollars for a five-dollar cab ride. He told me his daughter lived with his folks in San Francisco, but they paid for him to fly out once a month to see her.

I shook his hand so strongly through the pathetic little opened sliding partition and wished him good luck. We'd been double-parked, talking for at least ten minutes next to the curb of my building. What a blur the rest of the afternoon was for me. I played with John, fixed supper for him, bathed him and put him to bed. And all the while the glow of Drew's happy, warm face floated around me. How wonderful to know that there still was a man left in the world who loved me. And a call from Lizzie in London. She was pregnant! The baby due in August. It was as if good news of all kinds swirled around me.

The next day passed in a way long forgotten: a day of lingering and treasuring the details of the previous day. It was like being in love, and I, instead of backing away from this forgotten feeling, wanted to enjoy it. There was a sureness in the air, an expectancy. The telephone rang. "Nance, this is Drew. I'm at a party for a guy who's leaving the bank, and I know you write after John goes to bed at seven, but I was wondering if you'd like to do something else?"

That caught my breath and took it away in one big grateful leap. "I don't believe it," I kept repeating after I hung up the phone. What better, happier thing could happen to me on the eve of the day John was operated on two years before? Somehow it was almost as if John had arranged this, had seen to it all, that, yes, it was going to be Drew who'd be the first one, the first one to touch me in two years. It was probably more out of friendship than lust and maybe a touch of curiosity. He'd asked about it the previous day, and I had said, "No, no one, not in two years." And he'd said, "You mean you haven't made love in two years? Nobody's . . . ?" "That's right, Drew, nobody."

Drew arrived by ten. And what a grin he gave me, and I returned it to him as he came through the door into my home. We sat and talked on the couch for a while, probably not very long, and Drew reached out for my shoulder and pulled me toward him and hugged me so tightly. And cautiously, as if I didn't want to tear a precious document, I slowly raised my arms, my hands passing over the smooth material of his suit stretched across his back, and finally threw my arms around his neck. He understands, he understands, I thought to myself.

Afterward I lay with my head on his chest in my bed as he stroked my hair. I told him my fear that the first time a man held me I would start to cry and never be able to stop, but I said, "I don't feel like crying. I'm just happy." And Drew kidded me, and hugged me tighter as he said, "Gee, I at least expected tears!" By midnight he was gone. Back to his wife, back to his children.

The next morning I woke up still thinking about Drew.

How incredibly lonely I must have been, how longing for a man, but especially a friend. I thought I'd turned to ice all these long months, that only toward my little boy could I feel and show love. But here was Drew, the man who really put his arms around me. He had carried my phone number in his pocket all day. He had even gone to his office especially early to get it before heading for a meeting downtown. "I knew you needed me." I thought of his "Oh, Nancy, Nancy, what are we going to do?" Of his "I don't want to fuck up your life." And of my "Don't worry, Drew, I don't want to get married." "Yes," he said, "we've been through that before." "Yes," I said, "ten years ago." "Ten? Has it really been ten years? It just doesn't seem that long ago." I thought of his laughter, the way his smile put a skip in my feet that morning; he knew what I'd lost in John and he understood better than any of my other friends ever could.

But where had that night taken us? Where did we indeed go from there? I pushed my mind, as I washed John's and my breakfast dishes, to the razor edge of morality. Maybe his wife had said something like "I don't want to know who, but if you ever, so much as ever call her again . . ." And if Drew did in fact never call, I would understand why. He was not just a man who held me on a night I needed to be held; he was, after John, one of my best friends, and I was happy to let the night remain an island of joy.

All day long I thought and worried and struggled. Is this, I wondered, the difference between men and women: that if it had been Drew's wife instead of John who had died, and if Drew had needed me two years later as much as I needed him, the absolute fact is that I would not have slept with him? I might have had lunch with him, but as the wife of a living John Rossi, I would not have slept with him. And yet my feelings for Drew would have been the same as they were that morning, but without the

physical coupling. I suppose I would have done the comforting with words.

And to prove women's loyalty, or really my loyalty, yet
again, I thought, if even an old friend asked me to sleep
with him in the near future, I would not be able to. Because I'd slept with Drew I needed to resolve our future
before I could sleep with another. Just one lovemaking
makes me loyal unless I'm totally laughed at and betrayed.
I'm one of thousands of Penelopes.

That night I remember I went into John's room and
pulled the covers closer around him and held his soft,
sleepy hand. This was my life, to bring up my little boy.
Drew's life was his wife and his work. I ended that day-
dreaming day hoping he wouldn't call me the following
week as he'd said he would.

Drew did call the next week. He had just been notified
by his bank that he was being made the head of their London office. We laughed.

"I love you, kid, you know that. Listen, you're going to
be okay."

"I know, Drew, thank you. I love you, too."

About twice a year we talk on the phone.

CHAPTER ELEVEN

M y son and I didn't get out to Wyoming the summer of '81. We spent July and a lot of August in New York City. Since John's second January birthday, more and more of my time, in rushed, hectic spurts, had been taken up with phone calls, documents to be signed, names and places and doctors to be remembered, old hospital bills to be reviewed, rereading the two shopping bags full of condolence letters written to me after John died, and meetings with the South Carolina asbestos litigation lawyers.

It had been clear soon after John died that a lawsuit against Johns-Manville, the manufacturer of the asbestos that he had been exposed to so briefly during a two-week summer job when he was in college, would be handled either by my father-in-law or by my husband's law firm.

Together they agreed that I should be represented by
a law firm in South Carolina, which is part of a small
network of firms in the country representing asbestos-
exposure victims and their families. Our meetings became
more frequent. I'd be coming back from the park with
John, for instance, and the phone would ring. Terry
Richardson calling, he was in New York, could he stop by
and talk, ask me some questions, when was the exact day
that John was transferred from Columbia-Presbyterian
Hospital to Mt. Sinai, and the whole day would change. A
day I thought was not leaden with sadness and loss would
now become one where the details of death were discussed with numbing detachment.

Terry, with a headful of black curly hair, briefcases and
papers and a raincoat and a bag of chocolate-chip cookies
for my son under his arm, would fly into the apartment
and spread out his notes and papers as we sat on the
couch together. Sometimes I'd look at him, this busy, brilliant man, the same age as John would have been, and
listen to his soft Southern voice, and think to myself, I am
not here. This is someone else making a list with my pen
of people I would be calling, of the questions I would be
getting the answers to, of the medical records I would ask
to be forwarded; this cannot be the same person who saw
her life pass away as she sat looking at her husband's bony
back as he lay sleeping in his chrome-railed hospital bed.
This matter-of-fact woman, sitting with a lawyer, acting so
grown-up. What a false picture. There was no doubt I was
slipping away, although my attentive head continued to
nod and my hand kept writing. And I was smiling as Terry
told me more about South Carolina, how beautiful it was,
how someday I had to visit one of the seacoast resorts,
"We'll arrange it for you!"

As we discussed the weeks ahead, the depositions, the
testimony to be given by John's doctors, by the men he
worked with at the warehouse, I realized I hadn't felt that

despondent, desolate and detached from the world since
the first days and weeks after his death. That same sense
of unreality. Perhaps, Terry suggested, I should be present when Dr. Chahinian gave his testimony to the Manville lawyers at his deposition. I backed away, fleeing from
the suggestion, not that I wouldn't want to see that brave
warrior of the cancer ward again, but how could I, I
thought, go into that office again without being engulfed
by memories of the day I helped John into the elevator for
an appointment there?

There was something in the air. Only the day before
John's brother calling me, and Uncle Jack visiting us, and
then David Clark's call and my breaking down and saying
to him that I miss John so much and David saying that he
had just been thinking of him the other day and that soon
he'd start to cry, too. It made me feel we were all lost and
that no amount of litigation and money could make up for
the expansive blank space where John had occupied our
lives.

Of course this case had to be tried. It was important, but
I couldn't make the leap to belief that John's life was worth
only money now. Why did I agonize over the morals of
this, when the facts were real and unbearably shattered a
basic trust in America and the methods businesses use to
get that third-quarter profit? John and others are ghosts on
Johns-Manville's annual reports that force us, the lawyers,
the widows, the families, on to exposing the murderous
cover-up of asbestos. That it is not only lifetime workers in
construction or manufacturing work who die after years of
exposure, for it is known that even brief exposure to those
invisible particles that are inhaled red-circles a future day
of illness and death.

John, only two weeks of handling asbestos sheeting the
summer he was twenty; the little boy in Denver who died
after spending two days, proudly surely, with his father at
the factory Daddy worked in. And the management of

Johns-Manville suppressing what they knew, not warning anyone, not warning until they were forced to, then providing safety guidelines for those workers who handled it. How could it be that only sixteen years ago when John was hauling those sheets off the back of a truck, no one was told to wear even a surgical mask, the warehouses were not ventilated, and instead Johns-Manville repeatedly assured the world of the safety of the substance?

What, I was asked by a British film crew, who interviewed me for a documentary about asbestos a few weeks earlier, what would I say to the head of Johns-Manville if I met him today, and there I was sitting on a chair in my living room with microphone wires all through my blouse and skirt—"Just like we hook up the Queen Mum"—the hot film lights on me, the camera pointed at my face, and I thought fast: I thought I certainly wouldn't waste my time listing the well-known hazards of asbestos or call him a murderer or anything, no, and my lips started to move in answer and I lowered my eyes. I could hardly bear what I was hearing come out of my mouth, but I raised my head and looked directly at the camera and answered that I'd ask him if he had any advice on how to raise a two-year-old son by oneself. This is what I can't understand: the big CEO of Johns-Manville probably has children, maybe even grandchildren. He was for certain a little boy himself once, and is he now so preoccupied with that third-quarter balance sheet that he no longer thinks about life? Am I supposed to believe that when he reads the accounts of the trial he will be surprised and naive? It was when Terry and I talked about the fact that years ago, in the 1930s, people at Johns-Manville were already scared, knew they had to cover up and in fact falsified their own workers' chest X-rays—"You're clear, Mr. Smith. No, not a sign of disease," and Mr. Smith dies, he and his family having no idea why, another ghost to accompany the accountants' record-profit year—that my spine stiffened and springboarded for the fight. How long did Johns-Manville think death would slip workers away unnoticed?

The hot July days passed. Terry returned to New York with the other lawyers. They would pick me up in a cab and take me down to the Plaza Hotel to discuss the depositions taken that day. The Plaza? How could they know what that building has meant to me in my life? The doorman buzzed from downstairs—they're here. Terry came to the door, and we rode down in the elevator together and joined Ron Motley and his associate, Mike Thornton, the lawyer from New Hampshire, where the trial would be held. We jumped in the cab and the door closed. We were in a stop-and-go take-chances cab, and as he skidded us through the Fifth Avenue traffic, past the Metropolitan Museum and the zoo, the Plaza approaching, I wondered how I would get my leaden legs and body up those carpeted steps, through the revolving door. Ron made us laugh with his disbelief at how fast we were going and how he hated cab rides in New York. Our bodies bumped into each other with each screech of the brakes. Ron was right, this was one of the worst cab rides. But beneath our laughter I was remembering lunches and teas with my father at the Plaza when I was a little girl, always feeling so grown-up going to the ladies' room with the quarter Dad had given me to give to the attendant; lunches with my mother, when we were laden with shopping bags; Thanksgiving dinners there; a seventh-grade birthday slumber party I went to where five girls and I had a corner suite of rooms overlooking the park, how we heard Rex Harrison was staying down the hall and how we dared each other to run up and knock on his door and then dash back before he answered; my brother taking me there for drinks in the bar to celebrate my eighteenth birthday; a night of love when Drew impulsively decided we would spend the night there; John taking me to brunch there; my taking my little niece there for ice cream. I even know

the table where my father asked my mother to marry
him.

We got out of the cab and walked past the palms and gilt
back to the Oyster Bar, where we sat at a couple of tables
pushed together and ordered drinks. There was a man sitting at the next table all alone eating his dinner. Ron told
me what a pleasure it was to meet me finally. Yes, isn't she
great, I heard Mike and Terry say. I took a gulp of the
vodka and tonic in front of me and they began to review
Dr. Chahinian's testimony taken that day by the Johns-
Manville lawyer, recorded by the court reporter. They
were extremely pleased. Chahinian unequivocally stated
that John had died from asbestos.

And the most disconcerting thing was happening. It
had been so long since I'd been with a group of men, and
listening to these lawyers talk shop, answer my questions,
and tell anecdotes, I realized that I was having a good
time. It was too much to grasp. Talking about my dead
John and behaving as if we were all at a party. They mentioned how they wished I could have dinner with them,
but they realized I had to get back. They were going to try
some place in Chinatown. Ron groaned.

"Come on," said Mike, "New York is the only place
where you can get good Chinese food."

"God," Ron said, "the places Mike takes us to when
we're in New York."

I sat there still, knowing I had to leave or I'd be late for
the dinner I was supposed to go to, and I didn't move. I
wanted to stay with them, go to that Chinese restaurant
and hear more about their lives, more about what a brave,
wonderful woman I was, and how they all wished they'd
met John. How vividly I described him and what a great
guy he must have been, that everyone they'd talked to
said that. It was a gift to be sitting at this table with people
who wanted to hear about him.

But by now I really did have to leave. Terry took me out

to the front steps, summer tourists surrounding us, pink-sandaled preppy daughters from Memphis, all of them lined up for cabs. Our turn came, and he told the cab driver my address, paid for the ride, and I waved to him as the cab pulled away. The heavy, hot steam of the July night rested in the cab as we waited for the light to change but then blew in my face as we sped at forty miles an hour up Madison Avenue to home. I stared out the window, and the thought that came to mind was how lonely it was to sleep in a king-size bed by yourself.

The date of my own deposition came as a surprise. John and I were to leave for Utica to visit his grandparents, but instead the Rossis were coming to New York, as they too had to give their testimony. We met Terry and Mike again at the Plaza, the Rossis to talk to Mike and be briefed on the nature of the proceedings the next day, I to Terry's room to do the same thing. My testimony would be taken first at nine in the morning. He explained that Johns-Manville's lawyers would be there with a court reporter. I might call for a break in the questioning at any time. It would be best to answer questions directly with a yes, no, or an I don't know. We went over the day John was operated on, the results of the surgery, John's and my conversations, conversations with the doctors.

An hour later we finished and joined Mike and the Rossis. Mike was taking us to Gaylord's for dinner. It would have to be one of my husband's favorite Indian restaurants. We were walking in a restaurant that had known John's footsteps, and it was a battle of courage to hold on to my composure. I bummed one of my mother-in-law's cigarettes. In all the time over the past year and a half that I'd met with Terry and Mike they'd never seen me smoke. I explained I could go for weeks and months without one, but . . . but my explanation got lost, thank God, in the taking of menu orders. I looked at my mother- and father-in-law. They looked so nice that night, she in a turquoise suit with her blond-gray hair, and he more vivacious than I'd seen him since John's death. Oddly, again, we were all having a good time; only my mother-in-law's trembling hand as she reached for her water glass and my cigarette gave away the subterranean sadness we tried to keep from rising. At a time when I was not dealing at all well with my own parents, my continuous struggle to be independent often causing hurt feelings, I reached out to and felt more comfortable with my in-laws. We made plans for the next day, the details of arrival times. What is the Johns-Manville lawyer like? I asked. He's tough, but he won't be rough with you. He wouldn't dare be. God.

The next morning Terry and Mike and I walked into the suite Johns-Manville had rented in the hotel for the deposition. There was a long wood folding table in the center of the living room, the furniture pushed to the walls. A waiter was about to billow out a white tablecloth to cover it. The doorbell rang. It was another waiter with a cart of coffee, orange juice and a platter of Danish pastries. People pulled up chairs around the table and the court reporter set up her machine. Terry introduced me to her and to the young Johns-Manville lawyer. Robert Smith, the other lawyer, had yet to arrive. I went into the bathroom and drank some water. I closed the door and got some comfort from the familiar Plaza black-and-white tiles rimming the walls and the hotel's back-to-back "P" logo on the towels. Though feeling panic and fear rising within me, I told myself that really this shouldn't be so bad. I had been afraid we'd be in some fortieth-floor midtown office building's conference room. I blew my nose and brushed my hair.

As I came back into the living room, I saw a tall gray-haired man in a good-looking suit and a red-and-white-striped shirt, deeply tanned. He was annoyed and was saying, "I thought we were going to begin at ten o'clock, not nine." Terry quietly said, no, nine. The man threw off his suit jacket, steaming and pacing, hands and arms spread out to the air in theatrical exasperation. He called his secretary on the phone, hung up, and announced he was going to fire her as soon as he got back to his office because she screwed up on the time. Oh, dear. I quaked, but slowly it became clear to me that maybe he was behaving this way for a reason, to unnerve the rest of us. I was certain that this was not the first time this man had begun a deposition in this fashion. He looked as if he were about to throw something at someone. Jesus Christ, he said. He talked to Barbara, the court reporter, how'd she been. It was my first indication they knew each other, and Terry explained to me that she was the court reporter Smith always used. She was pretty, with dark-brown hair, a lot of it curling from the August humidity. Thank goodness the air conditioners worked and we were not in the Plaza of Fitzgerald's *Great Gatsby* with sweat pouring down our faces that summer morning. Barbara was very quick and funny with Smith; she obviously knew how to handle him. The poor child of a lawyer looked on bewildered and maybe intimidated by his senior's behavior. He was quiet the whole three hours I was there.

Smith's blustering was subsiding, and Terry got his attention. He was going to introduce me. Aside from Barbara, Smith's eyes really hadn't settled on any of the rest of us in the room yet, and the waiters were still coming in and out. Now he was flustered. This was a moment my lawyers had been waiting for. They seemed to think Smith would be in for a surprise, surprise perhaps at my round, young-looking face, I don't know, but Smith was momentarily subdued as we shook hands. He glanced at Barbara. Was she ready? Yes. Fingers already on the keys. She turned on the machine. We took our seats, Smith at one end of the table and I at the other.

It was very matter-of-fact. Yes sir, no sir, I answered. He asked me my name, my maiden name, my address. All the schools I went to. When John and I were married. 1974. Addresses of John's doctors. My employment record. At this point I was answering with restraint. He was somewhat mocking when he commented how easily I remembered addresses. But upon hearing that I graduated from and then later worked at Nightingale, he paused. "Do you know Emily Frosch?" he asked. Yes, she graduated last year. "What a girl," he said. "She's at college with my daughter. Her parents are my best friends."

From then on his tone of belligerence changed to that of a man having to get the job done. The questions were the same, but his voice was no longer edged with scorn. He asked about John, did he have annual checkups, did they include X-rays? (I don't know.) It was on X-rays, I learned later, that Johns-Manville would try to put the blame, not asbestos! He asked me many questions about John's life before I met him. Some I could answer—where he was born, where he went to school—but I didn't know the year he entered the Army Reserve; I only knew the year he got his discharge. He asked about John's work at Kelley Drye. Now I stupidly elaborated on how well regarded he was there.

When he asked me if John had become a partner, it was over an hour into the questioning, and that one question was too much. I began to cry. Yes, he had been voted a partner in the fall, but it was to take effect on January 1, 1979, and he—and my voice cracks—didn't live that long. It's what he worked for, I cry—the late nights, the weekends we'd gone down to the office together, and I'd typed up memos for him, the hours and skill he put into his work. I felt like shouting at this man, yes, he made it only to have everything taken away from him. I couldn't stop and remember myself saying, "No, I want to say this, it must be said," and I told Smith about the trust fund Kelley Drye had set up for my son, of the income they'd given me, of the John F. Rossi Memorial Tennis Trophy. This man was not going to leave that proceeding without hearing this.

We broke for a recess. I was in the bathroom again, wiping my face with Kleenex that got wet, ragged and torn with tears. Oh, Bunky, I mouthed to the shower curtain, help me! I hated them all in there. When I came out with a fistful of fresh Kleenex, Mike sat me down on the bed and put his arm around me. Was I all right? Yes. I could go back now. I would be okay. I was all right. You're doing fine, he said, just fine. Would you like anything? Some orange juice, I said. My mouth was drying up. He got some. It was fresh orange juice, and throughout the morning I drank glassfuls.

We went back to the table, and I sat down again. Okay, said Smith, we left off at John's partnership. He backtracked to my medical history. My pregnancy. Was it, he asked, my first pregnancy? No, I answered. John's and my first conception ended in an ectopic pregnancy in 1975. Other than that have you ever been pregnant before? A slimy question. Snooping around for a college abortion? No such luck, Smith. The infertility years are questioned. The tests, surgery, the final success. Who was the doctor? Richard Uscher. Another hour went by. Time had no meaning. His questions skipped from birth to death to birth. We were now at the point where the doctors had told me their goal was to keep John alive long enough to see the baby. Barbara's fingers had left her machine. I apologized, thinking I was talking too fast, that her fingers must be tired. She fluttered her fingers to her face, and I said I would speak more slowly. "It's not that," she said. "This, this has never happened to me before. It's . . ." and she couldn't talk, her hands were covering her face, and she left the room crying. Smith's mouth was open. We all were frozen in time. I, by the summer of '81, had become so accustomed to the facts, the fact that, yes, John and I had finally conceived, that he was diagnosed with meso-

thelioma in my sixth month of pregnancy, and that, no, he
didn't live to see the baby, that I'd forgotten what effect
this sentence had on people. I was dry-eyed this time. It
was someone else crying. Another recess.

Mike again sat with me. "You don't have to go back
right now," he said. He jabbed at the air that this was too
much. This young man, with a wife he adored, was gripping the side of the bed. Smith and his silent associate
were with Barbara. Had the Plaza ever heard such agony
in its walls? Lots of crying wives, husbands, mistresses,
sure, but a crying group of lawyers and a court reporter
and a numb widow? The building would never be the
same to me. Never, I thought then, would I ever go there
again. The special-treat times there of my youth had been
ruined. No, not ruined but saddened by the fact that I
hadn't known then, as the violinist came over to play
a special song for my father and me, his five-year-old
daughter, that as a woman I would be talking of death and
survival within those same halls. A five-year-old child in a
black velvet dress with a white lace collar, brightly shined
Mary Jane shoes, plain white socks, her blond hair hanging straight, holding on to her father's hand, guided to our
table by Victor in the Palm Court. People's heads turning.
What a *little* thing! She looks just like Eloise! And how I'd
beamed. What the hell had happened?

We resumed the deposition. Only a few more questions, Mrs. Rossi. And fifteen minutes later it was over.
Mike stayed behind waiting for Mr. Rossi; it was his turn
next. Terry and I left. Smith came to the door, took my
hand in his. "I wish," he said, "we'd met under different
circumstances." I told him please to say hi to Emily for me
when he saw her. And I looked right in his eyes and wondered how he could work for Johns-Manville.

A few days later, Lizzie's mother called me. Lizzie had
had a baby girl. Lizzie had returned to New York for the

last three months of her pregnancy so that she could be under the care of the infertility specialist who had treated her many times before. We talked later, and she asked me to bring John and to visit her and little Kate at her parents' home in Connecticut in a few weeks.

The day of our visit was a clear, cool, end-of-summer day. John was happy looking at picture books in his car seat while I drove. It had been years since I'd seen her parents' house, and I was not sure I'd recognize it, but I did and pulled into the driveway. As I lifted John out of his car seat, Lizzie was out of the house and on her way to greet us, the nurse following with Kate in her arms. Here we were, two mothers at last, and as she knelt down to say hello to John, I gently touched Kate's little hands and kissed her forehead. Then John peered down as I lifted him up to see Kate, and he said, "This is baby Kate. Hi, baby Kate." Lizzie and I smiled at each other, these two special children meeting each other for the first time.

While the nurse looked after Kate and John, Lizzie and I walked behind them and talked. Mostly it was details: she'd be leaving to go to her and Woody's new home in Rome, where he'd been transferred from London, in two weeks. She asked how the lawsuit was progressing. We secretly shared our pride that our children were so good-looking, that neither of us had ever thought our own looks were particularly great, an understatement, but that wasn't it a fine, shared, mother's secret that our children were beautiful. I appreciated Lizzie's bringing up John's father, how proud he would be, and her saying how often she and Woody had thought of me these past weeks, her not even having to say with words, just her eyes, that now with the birth of their own child, John's death seemed even more cruel.

Another car pulled up. Lizzie's own Nanny was here to see Kate, and while John said goodbye to Kate, Lizzie walked me to the car. It was hard to believe we had to go back to letter-writing after this visit. Lizzie was now "Aunt Lizzie" to John, and I had become "Aunt Nancy" to Kate.

A few weeks later, I heard from the lawyers that the trial was scheduled for December, December 1981. Oh, great, I thought, just around the anniversary of John's death. In December it was postponed until March. "These things happen," the lawyers told me. What they didn't tell me was how often. For the trial was postponed again to April, and then to June and then finally to August 2, 1982, and then once again to September 13, 1982, an absolutely final date, absolutely.

Over the past years I had thought about the moral question of whether money could compensate for the reckless killing of a life, but asbestos and Johns-Manville took someone away from me and my son. The rage I felt upon hearing the first time that Manville has known since the 1920s and 1930s of the lethal effect of asbestos and yet proclaimed innocence then and innocence now.

I had just had the shock of hearing on a newscast about new asbestos hazards in school buildings, in a state health office building that had to be evacuated and closed, and on and on. And a call: the pathologists at Mt. Sinai had proved, three and a half years later, a few weeks before the trial was to begin in September 1982, that the tissues taken from John's body at the autopsy were full of the fibers of Johns-Manville's "Flexboard": asbestos and portland cement. And that ironically the electron microscope that showed this to be a fact, the electron microscope at Mt. Sinai Hospital in New York City, was funded, donated, whatever you want to say, a third of it was paid for by Johns-Manville. It made me want to throw up. Does the Johns-Manville management feel they've done their duty to all who have died or may die in the future from exposure to their product by donating one-third of an electron microscope?

I'm not an alarmist, but it made me wonder, should I in the fall when my son enters his new nursery school, in a lovely old townhouse, should I go around with an asbestos inspector? And then the story that I'd forgotten until now, that when the lawsuit against Johns-Manville was just starting in 1979, it wasn't too much longer after that when it was discovered that the tissues taken from John's body at the operation at Columbia-Presbyterian, which also would have been useful in detecting the presence of "Flexboard" materials, had been lost. Yes, all one can do is take a deep breath and contemplate the reasons why and how those tissues might have been "lost."

So if it is money that talks in American business, the third-quarter profit, then yes, taking some of that profit away from them is the retaliation available to me. I felt during the early summer that I was ready and now very able to fight Johns-Manville's lies at that trial; others had to be protected. I had gotten everything arranged. John and I would drive up to New Hampshire, where the case was to be heard, on Saturday, September 10, get settled, and prepare for Monday's opening hearings.

The Johns-Manville management were also making their arrangements in the early summer, and, on August 26, 1982, they announced that they were filing for bankruptcy under Chapter XI of the 1978 Bankruptcy Laws. There would be no trial now. They were not insolvent but said that their figures showed that if lawsuits against them continued to be filed in great numbers, by the year 2000 they would be bankrupt. So, in effect, they were filing for bankruptcy based on their interpretation of the future financial status of their corporation, not of the present. Everyone agreed this was a dangerous precedent. Conveniently, however, their action halted all current lawsuits from coming to trial, and only after probably many years of legal wrangling will it be known whether or not the case of *Rossi v. Manville* will get its day in court.

The lawyers asked me to attend the first bankruptcy court hearing and to answer questions from the press there; I went in numbness, and later saw my face and heard my voice in the evening's television news. They asked me to be the spokesperson for all asbestos victims and their families, to appear on Cable News Network, to appear with one of them, Ron Motley, and with G. Earl Parker, Manville's attorney and PR man, on *Good Morning America* with David Hartman. I did both. *ABC Close-Up*, the documentary program, asked to film me for an updating of an asbestos documentary they did four years before. I agreed, and they filmed me and my son in our apartment. Soon to come would be an interview by a reporter from *The Guardian* while I was in London the following week doing the research on a future book. I do not know how often I can withstand repeating the facts of John's illness and death over and over again into microphones, into a television camera, into a reporter's notebook. Each future request by my lawyers to participate publicly in the outcry against Johns-Manville will have to be considered individually.

I take a deep breath and look at my husband's photographs that are still on my night table, and say, "John, you wouldn't believe it, never could you guess what is going on. But you know what, Bunky, you know what? You're not going to be forgotten."

NOVEMBER 1982